Teaching Hippocampal Anatomy

Teaching Hippocampal Anatomy

Edison K. Miyawaki, M.D.

Copyright © 2019 by Edison K. Miyawaki, M.D.

Library of Congress Control Number:		2019909686
ISBN:	Hardcover	978-1-7960-4649-6
	Softcover	978-1-7960-4648-9

All rights reserved. No part of this book may be reproduced or transmitted in any form or by any means, electronic or mechanical, including photocopying, recording, or by any information storage and retrieval system, without permission in writing from the copyright owner.

Any people depicted in stock imagery provided by Getty Images are models, and such images are being used for illustrative purposes only. Certain stock imagery © Getty Images.

Print information available on the last page.

Rev. date: 07/19/2019

To order additional copies of this book, contact:
Xlibris
1-888-795-4274
www.Xlibris.com
Orders@Xlibris.com

Contents

Chapter 1 Introduction 1
Chapter 2 Allo-, Archi-, Paleo- 5
Chapter 3 The Medial Edge of Cortex 13
Chapter 4 A Disingenuous Question? 21
Chapter 5 Alveus, Fimbria, Fornix 31
Chapter 6 Reverberation 37
Chapter 7 What's a "Place"? 45
Chapter 8 Grid and Place 51
Chapter 9 Medial Temporal Lobe, A Bit Magnified 59
Chapter 10 Negotiating a Triple Entente 65
Chapter 11 The Minimal Requirement 69
Chapter 12 More On Convergence 75
Chapter 13 A Parting List 81

References 85

1

Introduction

Neuroscientist R. R. Llinás has observed that there's a matter of scale whenever one attempts to explain anything about the nervous system.

Some parts of brain measure in centimeters; the adult human hippocampus—you can check for yourself in lab—is roughly four centimeters in length. The brain's largest individual neurons are visible with a decent magnifying glass, assuming good tissue preparation: the diameters of such cells are about one-tenth of a millimeter, or two orders of magnitude smaller than a centimeter. At the micron (0.001 mm) level of synapses between neurons, you need a good microscope to begin visualizing structures of interest. At six or more orders of magnitude less than a centimeter, you're in nanometer territory or the scale of trans-membrane receptors and their sub-parts.

"Most neuroscientists feel," Llinás writes (2001), "that two orders of magnitude above and below one's central focus is 'horizon enough,' and that anyone attempting four orders above and below is reckless."

It occurs to me that neuroanatomical education about the hippocampus is, in Llinás's lightly sardonic sense, reckless. In teaching that I've seen, we leap from gross anatomy into deep talk about memory and hippocampal long-term potentiation, the latter mechanism having to do with N-methyl-D-asparate receptors, which measure in nanometers. When we teach that way, teachers and students pass headlong across six, seven, or more orders of magnitude. That's a kind of exhilarating cliff dive, not without thrill.

I'm not so adventurous. What follows is intended for the interested and perhaps advanced neuroscience or medical student. I'll concentrate on structures that we can see either with the naked eye or with a standard microscope.

* * *

Consider the following magnified image, a coronal section. The stain (Nissl) allows us to visualize neurons:

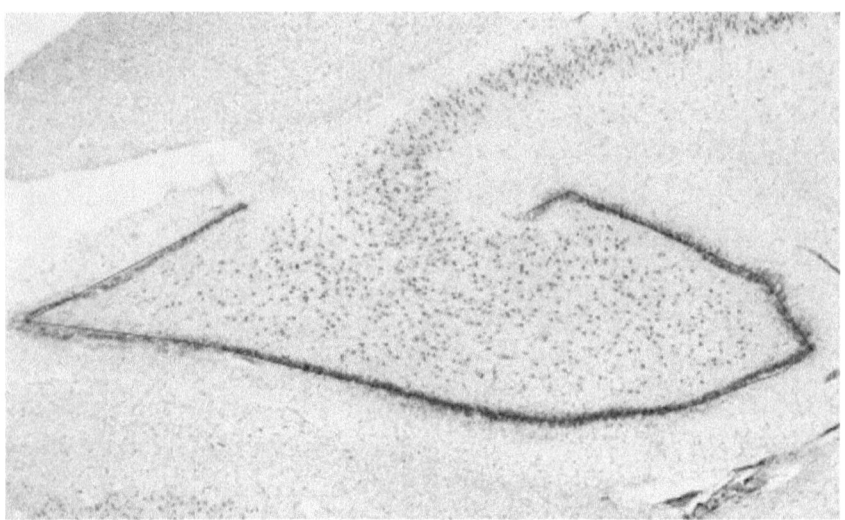

Resist a desire to identify parts right away.[1] Don't even name the general structure depicted, though the reader (clearly, an advanced student) knows what it is.

---

[1] Consider a medical student's testimony: "... learning new names for things is to learn new things about them. If you know the names of every tree[,] you look at trees differently. Otherwise they're trees. As soon as you know all the names for them they just become something different" (quoted in Good, 1993). I vote for looking, not naming.

Since the start of my teaching career, I've been curious about–and mystified by–the two convolutions in their unusual relationship to each other anatomically.

My eye is drawn first to the darkest black line that extends across the image from side to side. The ends on either side turn upward and inward on the left and right. Inside a kind of concavity thus created, there are many scattered dots (as visualized by the stain; we identify them as neurons, but there are other dots, too, that comprise the darkest black line–if those are neurons as well, are they the same kind of neurons?).

Inside the concavity, the scattered dots seem continuous with, and they apparently collect into, a neater, tighter band of dots to produce a curving swath that passes to the upper right hand corner of the image.

* * *

Those who study evolutionary developmental biology ("evo-devo" in the vernacular) observe that the structure in question is phylogenetically ancient (yes, it's the hippocampal "complex," which includes hippocampus "proper" [the scattered dots and swath] and dentate gyrus [the darkest black line][2]) (Li and Pleasure, 2014).

"Ancient" in evo-devo's contemporary idiom means that there are identifiable gene products that govern the development and maturation of the structure not only in humans, but also in other vertebrates in a highly conserved way, despite divergent evolution of species.

OK, so the hippocampus proper is . . . old.

Why should it be involved in memory in the first place?

Are there features of its development or basic anatomy that lend it to the task of remembering?

---

2   Amaral and Lavenex (2007) note that, after more than a century of study, there still isn't consensus regarding hippocampal anatomical nomenclature. In keeping with Li and Pleasure, I identify the hippocampal complex as stated.

2

Allo-, Archi-, Paleo-

Consulting my Carpenter and Sutin (1983), I find the following terms, all related to anatomy of interest to us; I'll list the structures alphabetically:

> allocortex or heterogenetic cortex
> archipallium
> paleopallium
> rhinencephalon

Paleopallium refers to something phylogenetically old (paleo), but the word "paleopallium" isn't at all synonymous with hippocampus.

"Archi" refers to something first (oldest) or perhaps *principal*, such as the "architect" of a structure. **Archipallium** refers to hippocampus.

Are allocortex (heterogenetic cortex) and rhinencephalon *not* old?

* * *

Here are practical definitions, taken from the textbook just mentioned, but with my editorialization:

Rhinencephalon = olfactory brain. The term rhinencephalon should be restricted to those structures that receive fibers from the olfactory bulb, namely the olfactory tract and striae, olfactory tubercle, amygdaloid complex, and parts of the pre-pyriform cortex.

So, what is **pre-pyriform cortex**? Follow the lateral olfactory stria towards the uncus on one side of the frontal undersurface of a brain: the **pyriform lobe** in that locale includes prepyriform cortex, periamygdaloid area, and entorhinal area. **Entorhinal area/cortex** projects to hippocampus.

Pyriform lobe also goes by the name of **primary olfactory cortex** (Haberly, 1998).

Paleopallium = rhincencephalon, provided that we apply the restricted sense of rhinencephalon just described.

Archipallium = hippocampus.

According to some, we should distinguish hippocampal *complex* and *proper* hippocampus from hippocampal *formation*. Let's address the differences one more time, just in terms of what we've already seen. The *complex* includes the **darkest black line** and the scattered dots that collect into **the swath** (*proper* hippocampus) that passes to the upper right hand corner. On the other hand, a hippocampal *formation* includes the complex itself and other structures to be identified when the time is right, not now.

Allocortex = the root "allo," like "hetero" in "heterogenetic cortex" refers to pallium or cortex *other* than neocortex. *"The allocortex consists in turn of archicortex and paleocortex. . . the pyriform cortex is paleocortical* [my italics]."

If the reader feels terminological overload, there's help at hand. Paleopallium/rhinencephalon as well as archipallium are old; allocortex is anything aside from new cortex. But distinctions still may not be clear: allo-, archi-, paleo-, and rhinencephalon ALL *are not* neocortex, right?

Oui, ja, yes, but . . .

* * *

For additional clarification, let's consult vertebrate neuroanatomy in non-humans (Northcutt, 1981). For example, those who study ray-finned fish, which amount to more than 90% of all known fish, don't talk about cortex at all. Their term for all of fish cortex is **pallium** or "a cloak."

The embryological development of archipallium in fish begins with a first/oldest thing situated above, dorsal to, everything else. In the following, I'll depict the two hemispheres early in fish embryonic life, in ridiculously schematic "coronal" section; each hemisphere has archipallium and pallium under it (the latter deep to the former):

```
ARCHIPALLIUM     ARCHIPALLIUM
   PALLIUM          PALLIUM
```

There are zones of pallium. For simplicity, we'll show just three; I'll call them "P1-3":

```
ARCHIPALLIUM     ARCHIPALLIUM
     P 3             P 3
     P 2             P 2
     P 1             P 1
```

In a process called eversion, for the fish embryo, it's as if the hemispheres splay open on either side, "rather like two tulips in a vase drooping away from each other" (quoted in Butler, 2017):

```
ARCHIPALLIUM                        ARCHIPALLIUM
        P 3                  P 3
            P 2          P 2
                P 1  P 1
```

The eversion continues to the point where the hemispheres turn inside out (P1 is rhinencephalon, which equals olfactory brain, which equals paleopallium):

```
                    P 1   P 1
            P 2           P 2
        P 3                   P 3
ARCHIPALLIUM                        ARCHIPALLIUM
```

Let's say that you're a goldfish in a rectangular shoe box of water with one (short) side in a different color from the other sides; the exit from the shoe box into open water is in one corner. If you lesion lateral pallium on both sides (the locations of archipallium) as opposed to medial pallium in goldfish, all post-surgical fish find their way out of the shoe box into open water, but fish with archipallial/lateral lesions have greater difficulty in the absence of the side with a different color (Vargas et al., 2006).

Fish lateral pallium is homologous to hippocampus in other vertebrates (Rodríguez et al., 2002), but I'm not sure what the shoe-box experiment says about archipallial function generally. And I'm even less sure, as astute biologists have observed previously (e.g., Butler, 2017), whether similar functions have anything necessarily to do with structural homology.

Mind you, the fish archipallium under a microscope looks nothing like the image in our first chapter. For one thing, there's no darkest black line—or anything that could be considered homologous to it, not in fish. And, in fish, there's no neocortex as we know it in humans, just (1.) olfactory-like pallium, (2.) limbic-like pallium, and (3.) other pallium linked to optic tectum and cerebellum (reviewed in Braford, 1995).

* * *

Let's consider how the developmental progression of archipallium in birds, reptiles, and mammals differs from that of fish. The start is the same (I'll abbreviate archipallium as "ARCHI-P"):

Teaching Hippocampal Anatomy

<pre>
    ARCHI-P   ARCHI-P
      P 3   P 3
      P 2   P 2
      P 1   P 1
</pre>

But there's no eversion. Rather, migration turns inward, towards the interhemispheric midline:

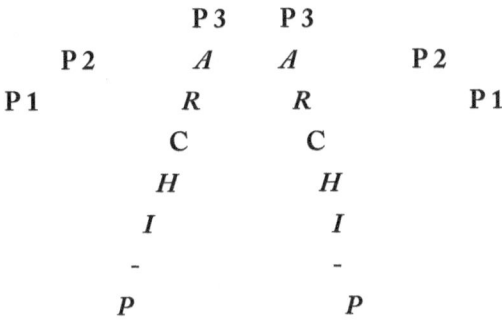

Archipallium becomes a medial structure. (P1 or rhinencephalon or olfactory brain or paleopallium is associated with archipallium, but they're not the same.)

If one coronally sectioned from front to back, one would demonstrate archipallium's presence over and again, always at the medial surface of the either hemisphere.

Wait, a student intones.

If she looks at an adult hemibrain (human) in her hand, she acknowledges obvious structures like **corpus callosum** and **cingulate gyrus** on the medial surface, but she's stymied by a request to identify archipallium.

Have her examine a 13-week-old fetal hemibrain (human), then her befuddlement should ease. "At 13 weeks, before formation of the corpus callosum, the entire hippocampal formation is visible on the medial surface of the cerebral hemisphere" (Kier et al., 1995). At 13 gestational weeks, rather than in the adult, there's neither a corpus callosum nor a cingulate gyrus, because neither has yet to develop fully. Instead, a thin band of cortex in the shape of a horseshoe encircles the primordial diencephalon.

Rather than a cingulate gyrus bounded superiorly by **cingulate sulcus** and inferiorly by **callosal sulcus**, the latter immediately above the thick interhemispheric corpus callosum in the adult, we have archipallium from front to back in the mid-sagittal plane. There's been hypercritical noise about whether a hippocampal sulcus exists in development (discussed in Humphrey, 1967), but let's admit that it exists in development. If so, then our student may confidently point to hippocampus, bounded superiorly by a **hippocampal fissure/sulcus**, on the medial surface of the early, pre-term human brain.

* * *

Based on his own animal work and with a nod to C. Judson Herrick, who worked decades before him, James W. Papez was quick to emphasize related and interconnected structures of what he called the brain's medial hemispheric *wall*: "It is generally recognized that in the brain of lower vertebrates the medial wall of the cerebral hemisphere is connected anatomically and integrated physiologically with the hypothalamus and that the lateral wall [think lateral surface of the hemibrain] is similarly related to the dorsal thalamus (Herrick). These fundamental relations are not only retained but greatly elaborated in the mammalian brain by the further development of the hippocampal formation and the gyrus cinguli in the medial wall and of the general cortex in the lateral wall of each cerebral hemisphere" (Papez, 1937a, reprinted 1995).

For me, Papez's importance (the pronunciation is "papes," not "pa-pezz," but correcting people has grown old over time) has more to do with the medial vs. lateral distinction than with his eponymous circuit. Elsewhere he writes about "cortical repercussions" that result or resonate from the activity of midline structures; in the same paper he talks about a "triple entente" between outer and inner environments and what organisms actually do in their lives (Papez, 1937b). Often in reading him, his terms seem fuzzy, but not in the manner of hand waving or intellectual evasion.

"Cortical repercussions," for example, deal with the emotional rather than mnemonic life, if the two are at all cleanly divisible, as I think Papez well knew they cannot be. A.R. Luria (1973) has noted that the first steps towards elucidating a circuitry specific to memory had been contemplated well before Papez, by one V.M. Bekhterev at the turn of the 20th century in particular, and he's perhaps correct. (One should also note, however, that Luria [1980], ever Russian, cites certain stories "by L.N. Tolstoi" as being useful in testing memory, but the stories trace to Aesop in antiquity.)

Whenever Papez uses the word "circuit" in his landmark paper (1937a), reliably there are qualifications: the circuit runs in two directions; you enter the circuit in different ways; there is always a "larger architectural mosaic of the brain."[3] A phrase like "mnemonic or emotional circuitry" is language that an electrical engineer might use, whereas Papez has us consider alternative "integrations"–not necessarily circuit-like wirings–relevant to what the brain *does in general*:

> ... the histories of the two walls of the hemispheres owe their disparity and distinctive structure to two different kinds of integration ... (Papez, 1937a).

---

3   From Papez (1937a) at his most succinct, with my emphases: "In this circuit impulses may be incited at two points: the cerebral cortex, and the hypothalamus. Incitations of cortical origin would pass first to the **hippocampal formation** and then down by way of the fornix to the **mamillary body**. From this they would pass upward through the **mamillothalamic tract**, or the **fasciculus of Vicq d'Azyr**, to the **anterior nuclei of thalamus** and thence by the medial thalamocortical radiation (in the cingulum) to the **cortex of the gyrus cinguli**."
I have a couple of incidental observations. 1. It's maddening that "mamillary," in my dictionary, is "mammillary," but the former spelling is everywhere in neuroanatomy; 2. A mnemonic for the circuit that I've used for years in my introductory courses has been "**MACH**," as in "Mach speed": **M**ammillary bodies, **A**nterior nuclei of thalamus, **C**ingulate gyrus, and **H**ippocampus.
The path depicted above by Papez runs in the opposite direction (H, C, A, M), but directionality isn't quite the point. A relationship between four midline structures is certainly the take-home.

You can download the paper yourself to decide what his two kinds are (speaking for myself, I'm not sure what to make of a difference between "hypothalamic" and "general sensory" integrations), but fundamentally and–I hope–not too simple mindedly, I'm curious to elaborate further on a history of the medial wall(s).

On either side of the interhemispheric fissure, I still wonder how the **darkest black line** and the scattered dots that collect into **the swath** passing to the upper right hand corner play out in that history–that is, how the distinctive relation of darkest line and swath hints at integration specific to the hippocampal complex.

3

The Medial Edge of Cortex

At some point in the mid-1990's, a senior colleague, who soon thereafter left Boston for a faculty position in the mid-western United States, to our loss, taught me that it reliably helps to look at any anatomic structure from more than one direction. Not everyone does, he noted laconically. If I did so with respect to the corpus callosum in the adult brain; if I looked at it *from the top down* in a whole brain in particular, peering at both the callosum's dorsal surface, I'd visualize, he said, items of interest.

Like a certain G.M. Lancisi, circa 1710 (Di Ieva, 2007), I'd notice (here I quote, with my emphases, from Nauta and Feirtag [1986]) that:

> ... a thin, inconspicuous sheet of hippocampal gray matter called the **indusium griseum** or the **supracallosal hippocampal rudiment** covers the upper–not the lower–surface of the callosum. It is positioned between the callosum and the overarching cingulate gyrus ...

Lancisi also observed two longitudinal striae that run from front to back, not from one hemisphere to the other, on the dorsal aspect of the corpus callosum. Those striae or "nerves of Lancisi" mark the boundaries of indusium griseum, the sliver of grey matter more or less literally placed upon the callosum's dorsal aspect (*induere*, a Latin verb, is "to put on").

If we considered the marsupial brain, Nauta and Feirtag observe, then we wouldn't have a corpus callosum with which to contend, since marsupials have just an anterior commissure and no callosum. So, perhaps one could study a marsupial brain, for the purpose of visualizing a hippocampus as fully as possible in its medial-surface aspect. An old textbook comes to our aid (Johnston, 1907, figure 160):

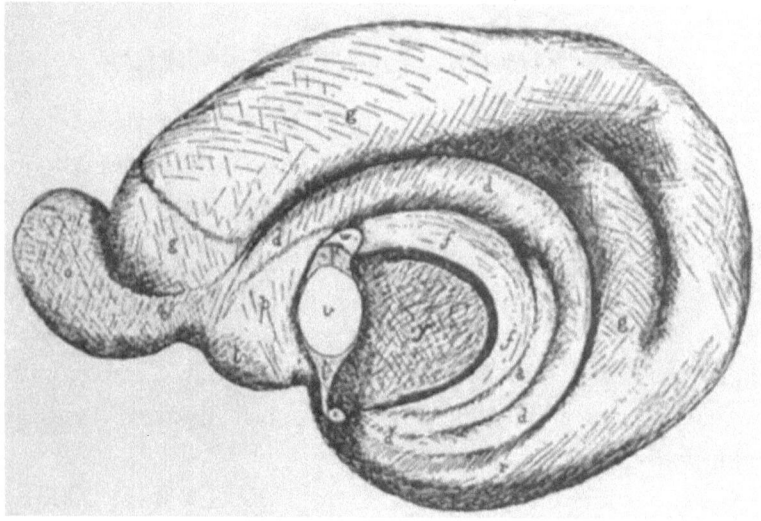

I provide a complete legend in a footnote,[4] but want, mainly, to note the arching, circumferential course of the structure marked "d".

Nauta and Feirtag trace much the same curving path in an adult human brain, now over and under a corpus callosum:

---

4   The drawing is a medial, mid-sagittal view of the right hemisphere in a marsupial. The front of the brain is to the left of the image.

Some individual letters in the figure are hard to see even in the original, but, regardless, the legend reads as follows: a = alveus; d = dentate gyrus; f = fimbria; g = neopallium; l = lamina terminalis; o = olfactory bulb; o´ = olfactory peduncle; p = precommissural body; r = pyriform lobe; t = tuberculum olfactorium; v = ventral (anterior) commissure; w = hippocampal commissure; x = optic chiasm; y = thalamus.

In its caudal extent, the hippocampal rudiment courses around the **splenium of the callosum**, where it takes on the shape of a slender, somewhat rounded band. Indeed, it becomes a miniature gyrus. In that form it extends ventralward, then forward, first on the underside of the splenium, then on the medial face of the temporal lobe as the **gyrus fasciolaris** or **fasciola cinerea**. (The second name means the little gray bundle.) Finally, it merges into the **dentate gyrus**, which caps the hippocampus and marks the true edge of the cerebral cortex. The dentate gyrus gets its name because a fairly regular spacing of transverse grooves makes it resemble a row of teeth. In its opposite, rostral extent, the hippocampal rudiment curves around the **genu of the corpus callosum**. Then, after following the underside of the rostrum, it descends vertically on the medial face of the cerebral hemisphere. In this last part of its course it is called the **taenia tecta**–the hidden (covered) band. What hides it is a shallow groove, the **sulcus paraolfactorius posterior**, which marks the border between the frontal cortex anterior to it and the subcortical tissue of the base of the septum behind it. The hippocampal rudiment marks throughout its extent the true edge of the cerebral cortex.

Likewise, structure "d" in the marsupial marks a medial edge or border between archipallium and the remainder of the neocortex or neopallium.

* * *

Contemporary histological study suggests that three layers characterize indusium griseum throughout fetal development in humans (Rasonja et al., 2019). Others have observed that all elements of the hippocampal formation can be identified in the indusium griseum (Wyss and Sripanidkulchai, 1983).

Actually, we've already encountered a three-layered structure in the form of what we've called "the darkest black line," which we'll examine now in detail, with a proviso that it's not clear that indusium griseum is just a rudimentary **dentate gyrus** or structure "d," even if the former merges into the latter as Nauta and Feirtag describe. And, if we look again at the 1907 figure, it would seem dentate gyrus is *a continuous thing* without need to specify an indusium, because there's no corpus callosum.

As we'll see, "three layers" may be an overcomplicated depiction of archipallium.

Here are two schematized views of the landscape depicted in our first chapter. In the second image (an enlargement of the left side of the first), I draw attention specifically to a **suprapyramidal blade** of **dentate gyrus**.

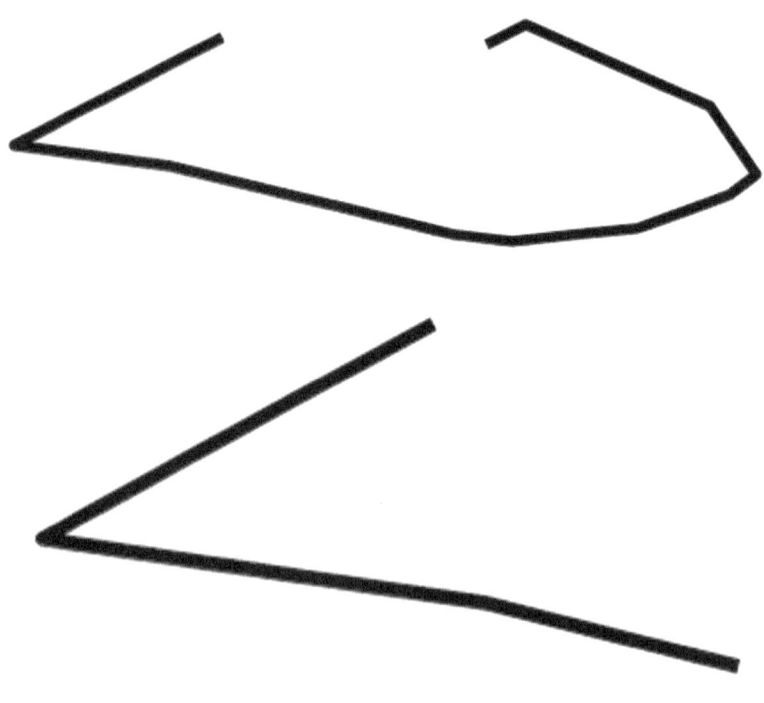

An acute angle is formed by the suprapyramidal blade and the rest of the darkest black line.

Textbooks and other official sources which blithely describe three layers of dentate in hippocampal complex make me think about three layers in a different anatomical structure that are more plainly visible. In cerebellar cortex, from pial surface on top to a densely packed bottom, we note a molecular layer with some cells in it, a Purkinje-cell layer (with monstrously large Purkinje cells in it), and a thickly populated granular-cell layer—all the above amounting to the three layers of cerebellar cortex.

Since many of the same anatomical words are used in describing both the dentate gyrus in hippocampal complex and the cerebellar cortex, it's worth acknowledging how different these two three-layered structures are.

In dentate gyrus, what we've called the darkest black line is the **granule cell layer**, which is positioned—as a middle stratum, not (as in cerebellar cortex) the deepest one—between a bland-appearing, superficial **molecular layer** and a **hilus** deep to granule cell layer. The hilus itself has parts—if you will, its own layers. Immediately below the dense granule cell layer (packed with its dentate granule neurons) is a **subgranular zone**, a unique region of brain where neurogenesis occurs even into late adulthood.[5] Deep to subgranular zone is a **polymorphic layer**, sometimes considered synonymous with "hilus."

In hippocampal dentate gyrus, granule cells have apical dendrites that pass towards the pial surface, with wide ramification in the molecular layer. But in addition, granule cells project axons via a **mossy-fiber pathway** to *deeper* points inside the concavity formed by the acute angle of the suprapyramidal blade.

---

5   Toni and Schindler (2016) ask a thought-provoking question about the subgranular zone: "Why is there neurogenesis in the dentate gyrus of the adult hippocampus and not in many other cortical regions of the mammalian brain with a high demand for plasticity?" The attention that we pay to the dentate gyrus and its granule cell layer in particular sets the stage for an attempt at our own answer.

In cerebellar three-layered cortex, on the other hand, granular neurons in the deepest of the three layers send mossy fibers *superficially* towards the cerebellum's molecular layer.

In the dentate polymorphic layer, interneurons called **mossy cells** are present, not to be confused with the aforementioned mossy-fiber pathway or, for that matter, the mossy fibers of cerebellum. In the deep polymorphic layer of dentate gyrus are **basket cells** as well; they're also interneurons.

By comparison, basket cells in cerebellar cortex are located in the superficial molecular cell layer.

* * *

The layers of dentate gyrus hardly seem obvious. One could argue that the gyrus consists of only one clearly cellular (granule cell) layer. Simplification helps: one could go so far as to say (Johnston and Amaral, 1998; Nauta and Feirtag, 1986) that the dentate gyrus is a single layer in essence. The same can be said of scattered neurons populating the concavity rimmed by the suprapyramidal blade(s), the general area indicated by the black arrow, below:

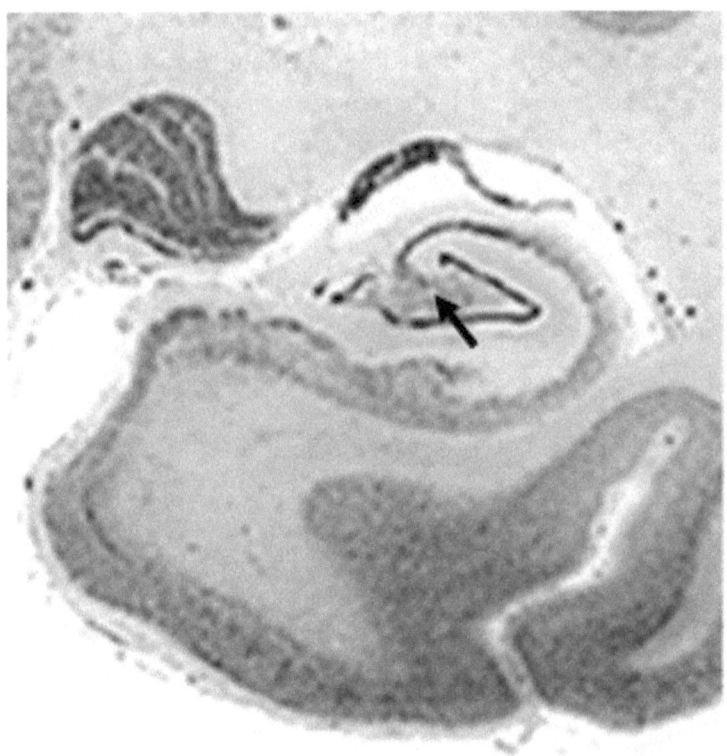

Cells in the vicinity of the arrowhead are **pyramidal neurons** which, as we've said, collect into a neater, tighter band, whose curving swath extends throughout the hippocampal *formation*.

Despite differences in their appearance, pyramidal neurons of the hippocampal complex and granule cells of the dentate could belong to the same category of pyramid-like neurons (Nieuwenhuys et al., 2008, p. 370 in particular). Pyramidal neurons are the main cellular constituents of **Cornu Ammonis (CA)** or **Ammon's horn**, whose parts we'll discuss in the next chapter, but we should observe now that precisely at the interface of the dentate gyrus and CA, we see two cellular monolayers, both archipallial, whose relationship is interesting if for no other reason than that neurogenesis and the production of dendrites and axons, even into adult life, occur in their vicinity.

Keep in mind, too, that the medial edge of cortex on either side is para-midline (think: "structure 'd" in the marsupial brain) and thus proximate to diencephalic structures as well as to brainstem in what Nieuwenhuys considered a vastly connected, midline "greater limbic system."

4

A Disingenuous Question?

I've cleared my desk to concentrate on a paper entitled "What is the mammalian dentate gyrus good for?" (Treves et al., 2008). The question is crafty, because it states a fact in the mode of an interrogative, that only mammals have a dentate gyrus. A few pages in, I read the following about "DG," which only mammals possess:

> The DG is one of a few regions in the mammalian brain in which neurogenesis continues to occur in adulthood. New granule cells are generated from dividing precursor cells located in the subgranular zone, the hilar border of the granule cell layer. Initially, extra numbers of new neurons are generated, and a substantial proportion of them dies before they fully mature. The survival or death of immature new neurons is affected by experience, including hippocampal-dependent learning.

Tracking down the reference in support of the first sentence (Gage, 2000), I find that a capacity for neurogenesis implicates neural stem cells, which can be harvested *in vitro* either from adult mammalian hippocampus (from the subgranular zone) or from subventricular zone deep to neocortex:

> The observation of stem cells in the adult nervous system has not been adequately integrated into our ideas of the function of the adult brain, which had long been thought to be entirely postmitotic. The importance of long-term, regular cellular self-renewal in the central nervous system is uncertain. In the absence of a defined function for these adult stem cells, it has been suggested that they are vestiges of evolution from more primitive organisms, like planaria or fish, in which organ and tissue self-renewal provides survival advantage in an inhospitable environment. An alternative view is that the adult mammalian nervous system retains a limited capacity for self-renewal that is important for its normal functions, like learning and memory. It is possible that the local generation of new neurons in structures could participate in the formation or integration of new memories.

Gage himself and, certainly, Treves et al. incline to the alternative view. Yet one wonders, if just for a moment, whether it could be mere coincidence that neurogenesis happens in hippocampus, a structure which, at least since Scoville and Milner (1957), had already been implicated and accepted to play a role in memory formation. Neurogenesis doesn't explain memory, not necessarily.

And here's a related concern: What really suffices to deem a particular structure important or quintessential in a higher cognitive function like memory? Since fish don't have dentate gyri (though fish have memory, about which we've learned a bit in chapter two), the question asked by Treves et al. becomes less than perfunctory.

We started this monograph by asking why hippocampus should be involved in memory at all. In my introduction, I intentionally didn't answer: "because lesions of hippocampus cause memory disturbances." Lesions in many locales cause memory deficits–the diversity would be the topic of a completely different monograph.

I've hinted that hippocampal connectivity is important by my descriptions of medial archipallium proximate to diencephalic structures and brainstem, both of which inform about the internal and external milieus, and by reference to Papez's medial wall.

We might be inclined to think that fish must have a memory mechanism involving a lateral archipallium; yet, as mentioned earlier, analogous function doesn't necessitate strict structural homology. Another way of saying the same thing is to observe that fish don't have a structure that mammals have (the dentate gyrus or DG), but memory of a kind is still possible for fish.

Frankly, is "because it's medial . . . or . . . connected" a decent response in an attempt to posit a specific role for hippocampus in memory? Neuroanatomy students for generations have lamented that most brain parts link hither and yon and yon to hither, so the word "connectivity" out of a teacher's mouth explains either everything emptily or nothing much at all.

It helps a lot to narrow our focus; I'll use the paper in front of me as my lens. More specifically, I want to obsess over this claim in the paper: "With the addition of new neurons the available set of granule cells is changed over time. If a given input pattern to the DG activated several newly added granule cells, the output pattern to CA3 would be different from one caused by a similar input pattern before the new granule cells were added." Are we reading about a model for memory in anatomical terms (changing populations of cells–change and cells, both of which we can visualize with little magnification)?

Before I launch my response, let me state the obvious, that *Teaching the Hippocampus* is an idiosyncratic approach; I'm writing a monograph, not a textbook. The format allows me to follow a line of thought, ideally with good pedagogical outcome.

* * *

Let's say that we'd like to trace specific connections in the life cycle of a dentate granule cell. Links transpire within millimeters.

By following the comings and goings of dendrites and axons, at very least, we'd learn additional, pertinent hippocampal anatomy.

The time frame of stem-cell growth seems extraordinarily fast.

Shortly after their birth, new neurons dispatch axons. *To where?* Within two weeks, apical dendritic spines of those neurons increase in size and number rapidly. By one month, the morphology of the new neurons is not unlike that of mature granule cells, but there's still dendritic growth.

Examine a gross specimen of hemibrain (right brain, adult, human) in horizontal or axial, not coronal section. We're at the level of the posterior commissure, which, along with a bit of right superior colliculus, is visible to the far left. There's some midline cerebellum, too, also to the left. The bottom of the picture is posterior; the top, anterior. I've drawn a black line that crosses from lateral geniculate body anteriorly into the hippocampal formation posteriorly.

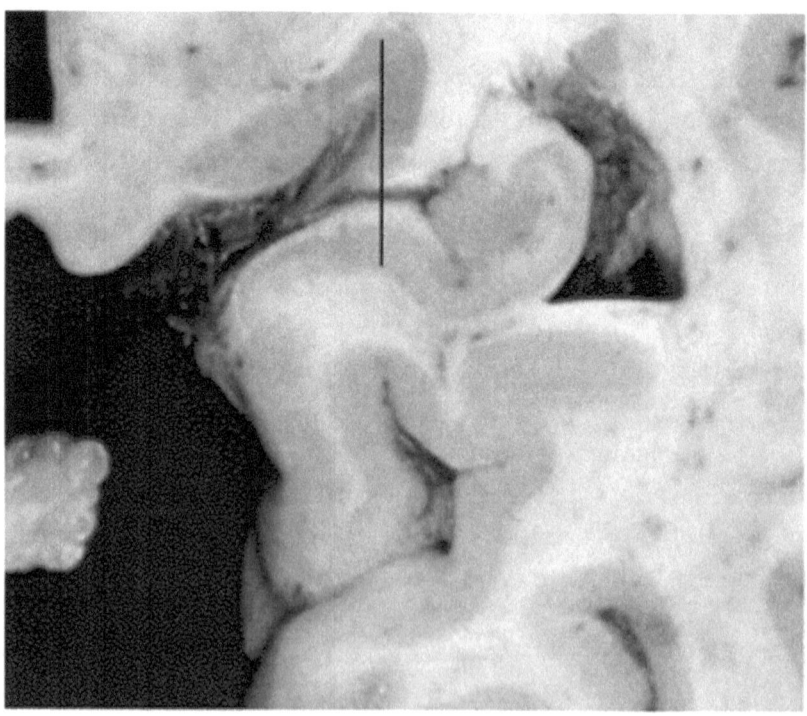

Specifically, exclusively, *new neuronal axons go from where to where?*

Axons that constitute a mossy-fiber pathway, arising from new neurons in the granule cell layer, pass to what Ramón y Cajal called *regio inferior*, a specific part of Cornu Ammonis otherwise known as **CA3**. Cajal also described a *regio superior*, considered equivalent to **CA1**.

Keep *unidirectional* travel from dentate gyrus *just* to CA3 in mind as we revert back to a coronal section, still in right brain (medial is still to the left of the image, lateral to the right side, as was the case in horizontal section), under magnification:

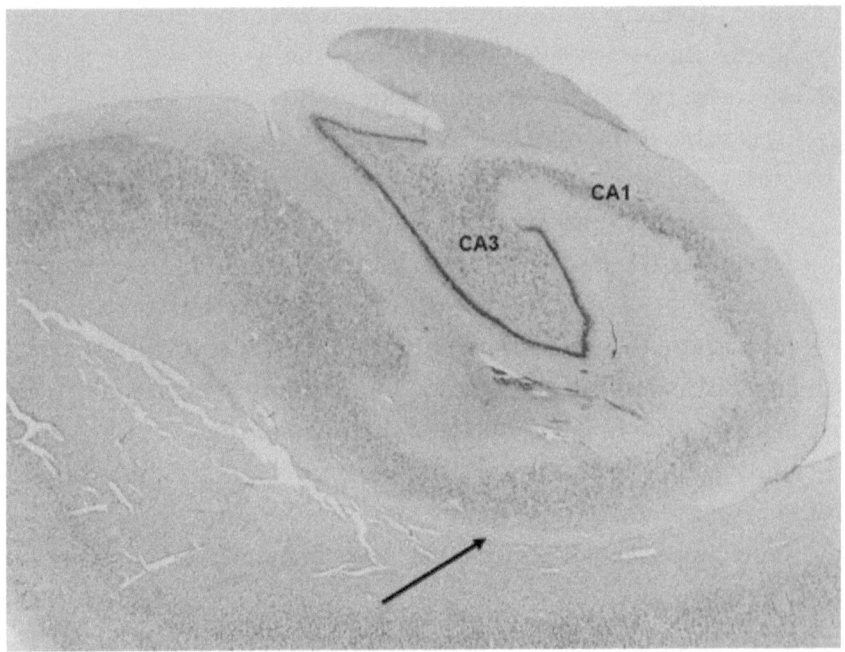

I've labeled the approximate locations of *regio inferior* (CA3) and *regio superior* (CA1). To determine the areas' precise boundaries would require a look at individual pyramidal cells in each area and their respective connections. CA3 neurons are larger than those in CA1; through life, CA3 neurons receive new mossy fiber input from dentate gyrus directly; CA1 neurons don't, not directly. For simplicity, I decline to label CA2 and CA4. The tip of black arrow is in the **hippocampal fissure/sulcus**, a potential space.

***

Does it seem strange to you (unique in the nervous system) that in the life of a new granule cell just outlined, axons go nowhere else aside from CA3? Isn't it also strange that input to new granule cells is also unidirectional? One way, but from where?

Recall the line drawn from the lateral geniculate body into the area of the hippocampal *formation*.

The dentate gyrus is *lateral* to the black line. I use the line through lateral geniculate body to separate **presubiculum** from subiculum (presubiculum to the medial side–to the left–of the line) in the curving swath that emerges from the lateral side of dentate gyrus. To the right of the line, posterior to (if you will, under) dentate gyrus, is **subiculum**, which literally looks to "support" hippocampal structures anterior to it.[6]

We're about to distinguish a number of structures all en route to identifying the place from which inputs into granule cell apical dendrites arise. **CA3, CA1, subiculum** are lateral to the line. **Presubiculum**, then **parasubiculum**, and, finally, **entorhinal cortex**, which is considered an anterior portion of **parahippocampal gyrus**, are medial to the line (moving lateral to medial from the line).

Only subiculum shares with CA3 and CA1 the histology of being essentially a cellular monolayer, and the entorhinal cortex "is the only hippocampal region that unambiguously demonstrates a multilaminar appearance" (Amaral and Lavenex, 2007; the authors have to be congratulated for their clarity, hence the direct quote). By "multilaminar," I'll add, we're talking six layers. In fact, Ramón y Cajal identified seven.

---

6   I borrow the trick of using lateral geniculate body from Nauta and Feirtag (1986), who go on to describe what distinguishes presubiculum from subiculum microscopically: "[under the lateral geniculate body] . . ., the presubiculum gives way to the subiculum, the first of a series of single-cell layered fields composing the hippocampus itself." Subiculum, like CA1 and CA3, could be considered a monolayer of neurons.

Not being a professional hippocampologist, all I want to emphasize here is that entorhinal cortex is the key (some summarize by saying "the only") source of projections that synapse on the apical dendrites of granule cells in the molecular layer of the dentate gyrus. Also, the visible extent of entorhinal cortex, at the most medial aspect of the temporal lobe, is marked by a rough pial surface giving the impression of warts or **entorhinal verrucae**, which have been studied in high-Tesla MRI reconstructions of normal brains and those with hippocampal pathology. Loss of the warts is associated with hippocampal pathology; normal aging produces *more* warts (Augustinack et al., 2012).

***

Some might say that I'm taking too much time describing a trisynaptic pathway that: a. is famously associated with the hippocampal formation; and b. is easy enough to memorize without need to discuss anything further.

Brodal (1981) talks about how the organization of the hippocampal formation is simpler than in neocortex, and that, accordingly, it's a favorable site for study, but he also warns, with greater validity today than when he wrote, that the organization is "after all rather complex." When the likes of a Brodal says "after all," we can surmise that the organization is so complex as to defy description, yet the organization begins with three connections in a unidirectional row. (Think about how pathways in neuroanatomy seem so simple at the start, like the three synapses involved in sensory information ascending to cortex in the spinothalamic and lemniscal pathways.)

Hippocampal connections strike me as extraordinary because of the route they traverse. To clarify:

Synapse 1: Entorhinal cortex, the only unambiguously six-layered structure in the hippocampal *formation* (more than complex) we now discuss, **to dentate gyrus** (molecular layer). More specifically, the origin in entorhinal cortex is layer II. Islands of cells in that layer are thought responsible for the surface warts, entorhinal verrucae, just mentioned. To arrive at the dentate, fibers must pass through parasubiculum, presubiculum, subiculum and then across hippocampal fissure/sulcus into the dentate gyrus, as has been elucidated in high-Tesla-MR tractography (Augustinack et al., 2010). The passage across the hippocampal fissure/sulcus–which is a virtual fissure in life–happens via the **perforant pathway**.

Synapse 2: **Granule cell layer** in dentate gyrus, via the mossy fiber pathway, **to regio inferior** otherwise known as **CA3**. Unidirectional connection is still our rule of thumb.

Synapse 3: *Regio inferior*, otherwise known as **CA3**, **to** *regio superior*, otherwise known as **CA1**. The connection to CA1 happens via so-called **Schaffer collaterals**. A Hungarian working about the same time as Cajal in Spain, Karl Schaffer's observations from 1892 about *very long axonal* connections between neighboring cortical fields (Andersen et al., 2007) should, I think, give us reason to rethink the trisynaptic pathway . . . for the simple reason that, after CA1, *there are other synapses*: specifically, **CA1 to subiculum** and **subiculum to entorhinal cortex**.

Notice that we've sketched a round trip from entorhinal cortex back to itself. The origin and terminus differ slightly: the trip starts in superficial layers of entorhinal cortex (layer II, maybe III, too), but ends in its deeper layers (layers V and VI). At the start of the circuitous route, CA3 doesn't project back to dentate; CA1 doesn't project back to CA3; and subiculum doesn't project back to CA1, but:

> Once one reaches CA1 and the subiculum, the pattern of intrinsic connections begins to become somewhat more elaborate. CA1, for example, projects not only to the subiculum but also to the entorhinal cortex. Furthermore, whereas the subiculum does project to the presubiculum and the parasubiculum, its more prominent cortical projection is directed to the entorhinal cortex (Amaral and Levenex, 2007).

***

Let's reintroduce that new neurons add to the granule cell layer throughout adult life.

Modify the dentate gyrus, and, presumably, CA3 changes downstream as a consequence. CA3 output, and then CA1 activity mediated by Schaffer collaterals, could each reflect: 1. the addition of any granule cells upstream in dentate gyrus; 2. the unique functional features of young versus mature granule cells, whatever the maturation of young granule cells itself entails.

Treves et al. wonder about an early, critical period: "1. The addition of new neurons (even if random) may enhance pattern separation in CA3 by providing additional available sets of input patterns. 2. Young new neurons may play a special role in memory encoding in CA3 because of their unique properties that mature neurons do not have. 3. The specific inclinations of new neurons, mediated by experiences during their critical period, may improve CA3 representations established after those new neurons mature. Obviously these are not mutually exclusive . . ."

***

Questions arise from the one seminal query: what *is* the mammalian dentate gyrus good for?

Why does six-layered cortex (entorhinal cortex) project to it only to receive connections back via the subiculum?

What's important about CA1 or subiculum or presubiculum or parasubiculum, as opposed to dentate gyrus?

What, then, about the vaunted Papez circuit that we all learn in medical school?

5

Alveus, Fimbria, Fornix

Have you noticed a particular anatomical relationship between the circled structure and what's deep/posterior to it?

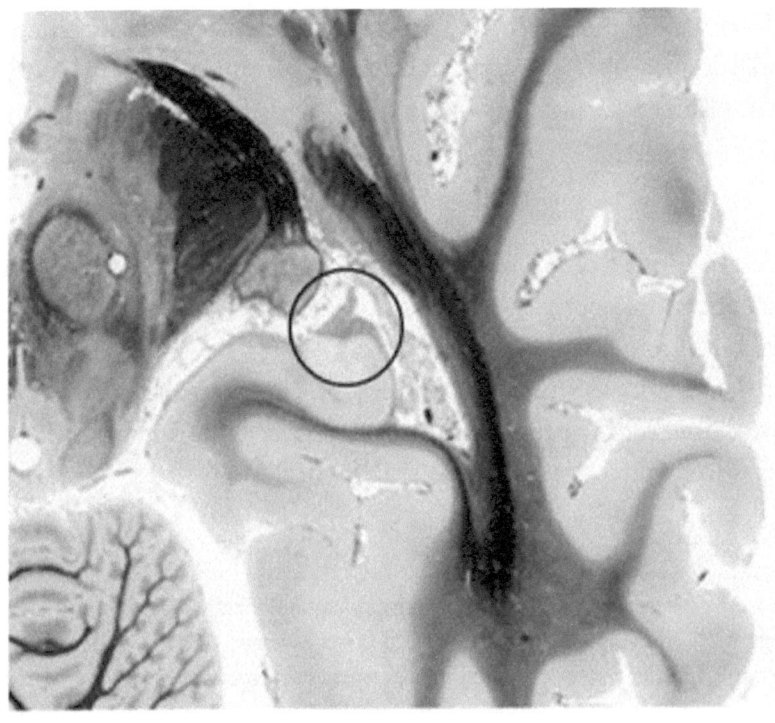

The circled structure is the **alveus** (a "belly," of a sort), which is composed by fibers that contribute to **fimbria fornicis** (the "fringe" of the fornix; a fimbria in a hemisphere enlarges as one passes from anterior to posterior brain); in turn, the **fornices**–each **fornix** in humans with about a million myelinated fibers in it, as many as are found in an optic tract–will "arch" their way upward and anteriorly, inferior to both the corpus callosum and septum pellucidum, eventually to descend in the direction of the anterior commissure.

As the fimbriae expand and fan posteriorly on either side, the fornices arising from them converge at the midline at a **fornical or hippocampal commissure**. In the rat, the interhemispheric connection is significant[7]; in humans, however, "there is almost no commissural interaction between the hippocampal formations on each side of the human brain" (Amaral and Lavenex, 2007).

Over the years, for me, alveus has been a useful, myelinated landmark: deep to it, I'd reliably find the vicinity of CA3 in relationship to dentate gyrus. Alveus marks the rostral hippocampus (rostral hippocampal *complex*). Alveus is anatomically contiguous with fimbria and fornix.

* * *

We can address projections via alveus/fimbria/fornix without fear or loathing. I'll excerpt a sketch that isn't shy about (oddly fascinating) details, but it remains concise.

In the vicinity of anterior commissure, the descending columns of fornix divide into **pre-commissural fornix** (anterior to anterior commissure) and **post-commissural fornix** (posterior to anterior

---

[7] Quoting work specifically in the rat, Brodal (1981) elaborates that "[c]*ommissural connections* between the two hippocampal formations are numerous. Tracings with silver impregnation methods . . . indicate that the *hippocampal commissure* contains partly connections between corresponding regions of the two hippocampal formations and partly heterotopic connections. For example, some fibers from the entorhinal area end in certain parts of the contralateral hippocampus proper."

commissure), each with a heady set of destinations, per O'Keefe and Nadel (1978a, my emphases):

> The pre-commissural fornix distributes to most of the **nuclei of the septal area**, including the **lateral septum**, the **diagonal band of Broca**, and the bed nucleus of the anterior commissure; fibers also terminate in the **nucleus accumbens septi** . . . Fibers traverse the septal region and continue into the **preoptic area** [of anterior hypothalamus] as the **fascicles of Zuckerkandel,** some terminating in the lateral pre-optic region while others turn caudally into the **medial forebrain bundle** to distribute to **lateral hypothalamus** as far caudal as the optic chiasm. . .
>
> The post-commissural fornix divides into two approximately equal components . . . one is destined for the **thalamus**, the other for the **mammillary bodies** [of posterior hypothalamus] and **rostral brain stem**. . . [T]he former, thalamic projection derives from the pre- and parasubiculum, while the latter, mammillary, projection derives from subiculum. . . The number of fibers in the post-commissural fornix before and after the thalamic component has split off has been assessed in several species . . . The numbers for rabbit, cat, and monkey are surprisingly similar [200,000 before the thalamic component split, 100,000 afterwards] and are about four to five times that seen in the rat. A huge increase is seen in humans, where there are about five times as many fibers as seen in monkeys. [Thalamic destinations vary among species, but anterior thalamic subnuclei–anteroventral and anteromedial–are targets in the rat and monkey.]. . . The other major input to the anterior nuclei of thalamus is from the mammillary bodies via the **mammillo-thalamic tract** (the **tract**

of Vicq d'Azyr) . . . [T]he **anterior thalamic nucleus** compares the outflow from the subiculum, pre-, and parasubiculum, but only after a transformation of the subicular output in the mammillary bodies. . .

The hypothalamic component of post-commissural fornix distributes its fibres almost entirely to the mammillary bodies . . . [these] in turn project to areas AV [anteroventral] and AM [anteromedial] in the thalamus via the mammillo-thalamic tract [of Vicq d'Azyr]. The other projection of this area is to the mid-brain via the **mammillo-*tegmental* tract.**

* * *

In light of what we learned in the previous chapter, we might be curious to know what specific parts of hippocampus produce axons in the fornices. It's not a query answered unequivocally, as excerpts from two authoritative sources attest:

> In CA3 a part of the fornix begins. In particular, the axons originating in CA3 join the alveus, and so become part of the fornix. Before that they give off collaterals (the so-called Schaffer collaterals), which distribute to CA1 and the subiculum. In turn CA1 and the subiculum contribute to the fornix (Nauta and Feirtag, 1986).

> Until 1975, it was generally accepted that the efferent fibers in the fornix originate from the pyramidal cells in the hippocampus proper. . . *[M]ost of the fibers of the fornix are not*, as believed for some 100 years, *derived from the hippocampus proper, but from the subiculum* (Brodal, 1981, his italics).

If CA3, CA1, and subiculum all contribute to fornix, then there are multiple portals of egress from hippocampus. Axons destined for alveus/fimbria/fornix don't head to entorhinal cortex.

If, on the other hand, subiculum is the preeminent or only portal of egress from hippocampus, then axons pivot from a point downstream to CA1 to enter alveus/fibria/fornix. Those, too, would be axons that don't head to entorhinal cortex.

I've said it a million times in class, with abiding deference to Papez, that the fornix is the prominent output pathway from hippocampus, because it's via fornix that we get to rostral locales (e.g., not only mammillary bodies in hypothalamus and anterior nucleus of thalamus, but also areas that *aren't* specifically named in the Papez or "MACH" circuit as I've taught it in class, such as septal structures or the nucleus accumbens). It's basically true, by the way: fornix *is* a prominent output pathway from hippocampus.

But it's not the only output pathway.

So curious: alveus/fimbria/fornix diverts attention from the other, obvious thing that makes the hippocampus such an unusual structure in neuroanatomy.

A major output from hippocampus, via subiculum, is to the very structure that inputs so strongly to dentate gyrus: entorhinal cortex, its medial temporal surface studded with warts.

6

Reverberation

We've traced the following, specifically within the hippocampal formation:

> **entorhinal** (six-layered) **cortex** TO **dentate gyrus** TO **CA3** TO **CA1**;
> **CA1** BOTH TO **subiculum** and TO **entorhinal cortex**.

Let's add that each stop in the circuit (dentate, CA3, CA1, and subiculum) also receives direct input from entorhinal cortex via the **perforant pathway.**

The anatomy describes, overall, a feed-forward design with built-in redundancies.

Let's solicit textbook help again (with commentary, in brackets); I think the authors are especially helpful when they speak "at the global level":

> . . . the dentate gyrus and the CA3 field of the hippocampus do not project back to the entorhinal cortex. [KNEW THAT.]
>
> Thus the recipients of the layer II projection do not have any direct influence over the activities of the

entorhinal cortex. It is only after the layer II and layer III projection systems are combined in CA1 and the subiculum that return projections to the entorhinal cortex are generated. [FAIR ENOUGH.]

The return projections mainly terminate in the deep layers (V and VI) [of entorhinal cortex] . . . [OK]

The important point about these return projections is that they are exactly in register (i.e., they are point-to-point reciprocal [topographically organized from CA1 and subiculum to entorhinal cortex]) . . . [WE'RE NOT UNFAMILIAR WITH TOPOGRAPHY IN THE NERVOUS SYSTEM. HOMUNCULAR TOPOGRAPHY IS ONE EXAMPLE.]

Thus, at the global level, all of the circuitry is available for reverberatory circuits to be established through the loop, starting and ending at the entorhinal cortex (Amaral and Levenex, 2007).

A dictionary definition for "reverberate" is "to reflect repeatedly."

* * *

For the student who has patiently endured this monograph, we're at a place where we can characterize redundancy implicit in all that we've been discussing. The generous reader acknowledges that I don't refer to a tendency to repeat myself. Instead, she might recall three principal examples of redundancy in hippocampal organization:

1. It's by no means clear what neurogenesis in the granule cell layer of dentate gyrus quite means (Aimone et al., 2011), but we *regrow* connections between dentate and CA3 in life–so much we do know.

Dentate and CA3 may not reverberate *per se* with entorhinal cortex, but there's repletion or dynamic rejuvenation even at the start of the intrinsic hippocampal circuit (McAvoy et al., 2016), presumably always based on entorhinal input at the level of the apical dendrites of old and new granule cells.

It's a recurring process, redundant over time.

2. CA1 and subiculum reverberate with entorhinal cortex.

What about presubiculum and parasubiculum? In the last chapter, there was a nuance regarding postcommissural fornix worth reconsidering here. Half of postcommissural fibers head for anterior nucleus of thalamus, the other half to mammillary bodies.

The former pathway includes axons from **presubiculum** and **parasubiculum**. The latter pathway, to mammillary bodies, eventually projects back to anterior nucleus via the mammillo-thalamic tract or the tract of Vicq d'Azyr.

Regarding hypothalamus, O'Keefe and Nadel (1978a) observe that hippocampus doesn't project to the mammillary bodies directly, but does so by way of the subiculum. If, the authors go on to ask, one has the freedom of traversing several synapses (sometimes, five or more), is the exercise of tracing pathways really profitable? Maybe not, but we still rehearse recursions, specifically:

> a. Presubiculum (whose dorsal aspect is sometimes called **postsubiculum**) and parasubiculum both project to and receive afferents from anterior nucleus of thalamus (Amaral and Levenex, 2007) in the manner of a thalamocortical loop; b. subiculum, with its connections to and from mammillary bodies, isn't independent of anterior thalamus, since mammillary bodies and anterior nucleus of thalamus are linked; and, for your further information, c. both presubiculum and parasubiculum project to entorhinal cortex, so they both contribute like *kibitzers* to the

reverberative interaction of entorhinal cortex with CA1 and subiculum.[8]

3. Papez's medial wall was all about cortical "repercussions," about which we might now add a consideration with several "if's" and one "then."

If intrinsic hippocampal circuitry begins and ends with the entorhinal cortex; and

... *if* entorhinal cortex is an interface between widespread neocortical locales and the hippocampal formation (Insausti and Amaral, 2008); and

... *if* Papez-like triple entente is the abstract/fuzzy goal (iterative comparison of internal and milieus against what an animal does in the world),

... *then* wouldn't we expect that many structures–mainly medial ones, including those that we haven't broached–redundantly connect through the hippocampal formation and/or other structures of the medial wall?

To me, as an obsessive sort, the recursions, redundancies, reverberations, and loops all strike me as subspecies of a checking-and-rechecking mechanism. Many might object to the anthropomorphism: I describe hippocampal function based on what I can't help doing, alas, so much in my personal life. But so it seems to me. Anatomically, components of hippocampal formation seem arranged for compulsive reentry or what has been termed strong back-coupling (Hopfield, 1982).

---

8   One should add, parasubiculum *especially* projects to dentate gyrus: "A fact that has not been generally appreciated is that the parasubiculum gives rise to a fairly substantial projection to the molecular layer of the dentate gyrus. Like the lighter projection from the presubiculum, this projection occupies the superficial two-thirds of the molecular layer ... and the fibers have a predominantly radial orientation. Because the parasubiculum receives a projection from the anterior thalamic nuclei, its projection to the molecular layer provides a route by which thalamic input might influence the very early stages of hippocampal information processing" (Amaral and Levenex, 2007).

***

Gurus of the contemporary connectome dash in where angels, students, and especially teachers fear to tread. But I can borrow from my colleagues (Edlow et al., 2016) to imagine a way of thinking about many untold (but still likely reciprocal) connections. Just take brainstem locales as an example—A in midbrain, B in pons, C and D in medulla:

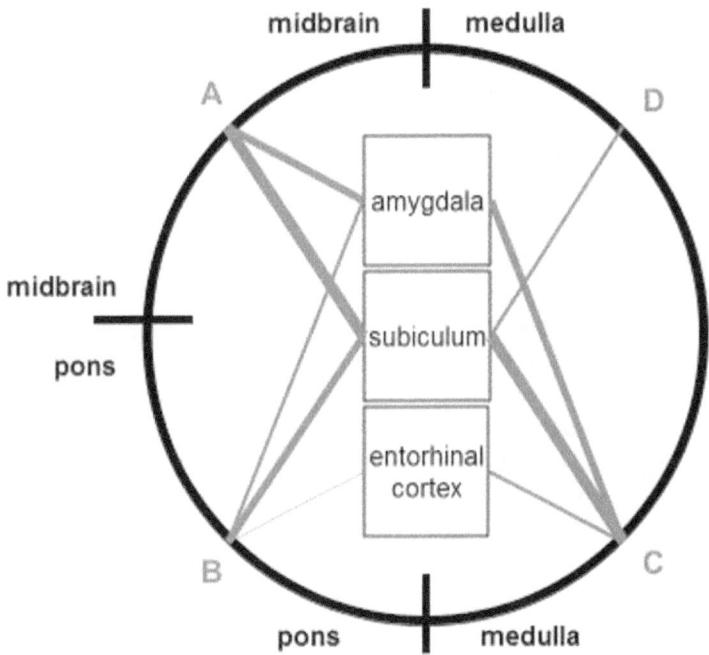

Thickness of the grey lines—what the authors call "streamlines"—indicates robustness of connections. You could add many other structures to the middle of the circle (other areas within hippocampal formation, for example); I've only chosen three—although the amygdala isn't technically part of the hippocampal formation.

You could conceive a different outer circle not having to do with brainstem at all, but rather, with paleopallium, cingulate gyrus, retrospenial cortex, and the parahippocampal gyrus beyond entorhinal cortex—what altogether was once described as *le grand lobe de l'ourlet* or the great lobe of the hem, visible on the medial surface of a hemibrain.[9]

Inside the outer circle, you could wonder about links between amygdala and/or subiculum and/or entorhinal cortex. It should come as absolutely no surprise that they exist. Hippocampologists and even basic textbooks study and debate them.[10]

"Bottom-up" and "top-down" signaling happens between brainstem and midline sites in the telencephalon: tractography doesn't specify direction. For our purposes, we might just think

---

9   Pierre Paul Broca eventually changed the moniker to *le grand lobe limbique* (limbus = edge). The history lesson comes from Nauta and Feirtag (1986).

10 For the record, I've taught in class that amygdala connects to entorhinal cortex by a route *different from* two pathways routinely associated with the amygdala. Those two common associations are the **stria terminalis** (amygdala to and from septal nuclei and hypothalamus) and a **ventral amygdalo"fugal" pathway** ("fugal" in warning quotation marks, because fibers pass *to as well as from* amygdala and diverse basal forebrain structures, including **rhinencephalon** and ventral striatum and pallidum). By a route distinct from those two, there are point-to-point interconnections between amygdala and entorhinal cortex, or so I've taught (using Nolte, 1999 as my source).

By comparison, read the following from Nauta and Feirtag (1986, my italics): "All the senses represented in neocortex–vision, hearing, and somatic sense–direct part of their traffic toward either or both of two cortical districts: the frontal association cortex and the inferior temporal association cortex. . . *In turn, the inferior temporal cortex projects to the entorhinal area.* The entorhinal area is the *cortical gateway* to the hippocampus. In addition, the inferior temporal cortex projects to the amygdala. In fact in primates it gives the amygdala its single most massive input. The projection is reciprocated. Indeed, the amygdala directs its cortical projections to the inferior temporal cortex and to the frontal cortex (specifically the orbital surface of the frontal cortex). It projects, therefore, to the parts of the neocortex in which the final stages in the cascade of sensory data toward the limbic system are embodied. *Evidently the amygdala screens its neocortical input.*" In the last sentence, the referent for "its" is either "amygdala" (which screens its own incoming cortical input) or "limbic system"–i.e., amygdala, in its reciprocal interconnection especially with inferior temporal cortex, screens cortical information which passes to entorhinal cortex in particular.

Is the direct connection amygdala-to-hippocampal formation as important as the intermediary role played by both amygdala and entorhinal cortex? My guess is that the latter role matters most.

about the bidirectionality in any "streamline," and reflect on the (very high?) probability that in any reciprocal connection there's functional significance. Other roundabouts elsewhere in the brain, across multiple synapses, invite the same consideration, as in the loops that connect frontal-lobe locations precisely back to themselves via structures of the basal ganglia.

* * *

Relevant to a basic understanding (again, just for our own purposes), Edlow et al. offer an important caution. A limitation that might be unavoidable in their tractography-based work has to do with the fact that axonal pathways traveling very close to each other may "jump" connections from one pathway to the other in connectome reconstructions. The result could be false positive streamlines, in the same way that multiple synaptic pathways can produce the false impression that everything related hippocampus starts and ends in hippocampus (or entorhinal cortex, or what have you).

The risk exists, one must admit.

7

What's a "Place"?

I'll simplify an experiment to illustrate an idea of "place" (O'Keefe and Nadel, 1975).

We'll require a counterpoint to "place" which we'll call "cue."

The question put to a thirsty test subject (a water-deprived rat) is: where is access to water in a given territory? I'll identify potential water sources in various locations in a box; "W" marks where the water really is:

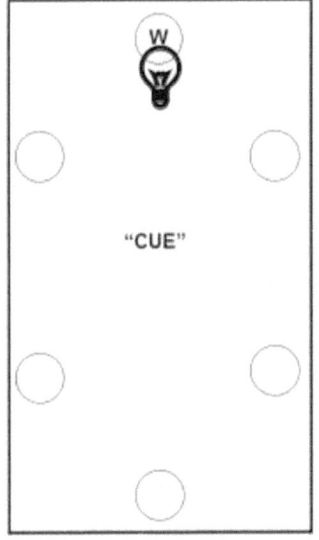
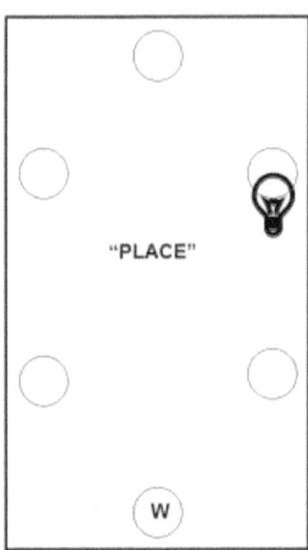

In a "cue" condition, a light always indicates the location of the water source. As illustrated (left box), light and water are due north.

In the "place" condition (right box), the light is an irrelevant stimulus, because access to water will always be found due south.

From chapter before last (though the point was fleeting) recall that in the rat, the hippocampal commissure contains significant numbers of fibers that interconnect hippocampi on either side–such is not the case in humans.

The experimenters created lesions at the level of hippocampal commissure using jeweler's forceps to crush fibers.[11] Lesioned rats were compared to control animals who underwent sham surgeries, including introduction of the jeweler's forceps into the skull, but without crushing fibers.

Lesioned rats learned the light cue very quickly, as did the control animals–in fact, the lesioned rats did a bit better than controls in the cue box. Controls also learned quickly in the place box: without hesitation after a few trials, they approached the source of water due south.

But the behavior of lesioned rats was different in the place box. They adopted a strategy of checking in all directions regardless of the light's location, and they didn't promptly glean the southern position of water trial after trial, with both an obvious and statistically significant difference when compared to controls.

The experiment followed a prior study (O'Keefe and Dostrovsky, 1971) which found increased firing of specific hippocampal cells in CA1 when a freely moving rat passed a particular position of

---

[11] Elsewhere, the same authors ask a good question, and they admit to the simplification in their 1975 protocol: "What can presently be said about the specific functions of segments of the hippocampus? The first thing that must be said is that much of our discussion is going to be simplified; we shall treat dorsal and ventral, anterior and posterior, lesions as the same, though it is clear that these are not equivalent in all respects. More pertinent, it now seems certain that fornix lesions [e.g., at the level of the hippocampal commissure] cannot be treated as equivalent to hippocampal lesions, while neither is the same as entorhinal damage. However, there is enough commonality in all these lesions to allow us the assumption of a unitary system" (O'Keefe and Nadel, 1978b).

space. The purpose of lesioning was to determine whether damage to efferent and afferent hippocampal fibers would affect the ability to discern/learn an outside location invested with significance.

The authors concluded that lesioned animals had a deficit of spatial, but not cue, learning. Fueled by the 1975 results, along with their 1971 findings, they wrote a review that morphed into a thickish book (their inspiration described in O'Keefe, 2007; the 1978 book is still available in 2019 at www.cognitivemap.net).

* * *

An interested student can pull both the 1971 and 1975 papers just mentioned, or perhaps she'd prefer to download *The Hippocampus as a Cognitive Map* and read *in* it.

She could assiduously read the entire book, of course, but gazing *in* it, just one flip after the title page, might suffice. There, in the dedication, she finds Donald Hebb's name.

Here's what I did with my electronic copy of the book: I PDF-searched "Hebb" in all 570 pages to track down when he's cited and how he's used by the authors. There are surprisingly few Hebb references, but that's no matter. Hebb at his seminal best (1938a and 1938b) is worth a peek. He informs both the 1971 and 1975 papers regarding "place."

We'll get to 1938 in a moment.

* * *

First, some background.

Historian Alison Winter (2012) synopsizes the career of Karl Lashley, in whose Boston lab Hebb worked in 1938:

> Karl Lashley had spent the 1930's and 1940's first at the University of Chicago and then at Harvard in pursuit of what he called the "engram"–a physical location and structure embodying discrete memories.

> Lashley trained rats in mazes, then tried to destroy their memories surgically. It was a total failure.

The dates are off. Lashley first worked and published in Baltimore at Johns Hopkins roughly in 1912. In 1950, reflecting on his preceding four decades (he retired in 1955, then died in France in 1958), he announced that "there are no special cells reserved for special memories" (quoted in Boring, 1960).

I think Lashley is appropriately skeptical about what today we'd call a "grandmother cell," whose action potentials fire exclusively on seeing images of one's own grandmother.[12] Memory of a discrete datum–*the* light in a cue box, *the* south in a place box, or my mother's mother physiognomy and no one else's–isn't monocellular.

Here's Hebb (1949, reprint 2002), thinking about the implications of "no special cells reserved for special memories":

> Lashley has concluded that a learned discrimination is not based on the excitation of any particular neural cells. . . If it is really unimportant in what tissues a sensory excitation takes place, one finds it hard to understand how repeated sensations can reinforce one another, with the lasting effect we call learning or memory. It might be supposed that the mnemonic trace is a lasting pattern of reverberatory activity without fixed locus, like some cloud formations or an eddy in a millpond.

---

12 Martha Farah (1990) articulates the skepticism: "Doesn't the existence of face-selective neurons, including neurons selective for particular faces, imply that the visual system uses extremely local representations for face recognition? No, because although these cells respond more to one face than another, there is a range of faces to which they will respond, and conversely, a given face will evoke responses of varying degrees in a large number of neurons. In other words, within the domain of face representation at least, the results of single unit recordings imply that distributed representations are being used."

Absence of a fixed locus, in fact, is a problem to a physiologist. She experiences consternation about an event in the absence of all context or a reverberation in unspecified anatomical space.

A few pages later, Hebb complains, "We do *not* know that pattern [cloud formations, an eddy] is everything, locus nothing."

* * *

It's ghoulish, but if you were to thermocoagulate up to 40% of neocortex (known as isocortex) in a rat, or blind another rat by enucleation, then compare either's ability to find food to what a normal rat can do, what differences accrue?

In 1938, Hebb found that cortical destruction didn't impede an ability to locate food in a certain remembered place. Even the blinded rat, like both the one with thermocoagulated cortex and the control, went first to the place where food once had been. Hebb later (1949, reprint 2002) reflected on his experiments in Lashley's lab in 1938: "And why is the position habit so persistent? The answer seems to be that the animal mainly perceives, and responds to the least variable objects in his environment . . ."

A search for invariance could be at play in the experiment that started this chapter, but that protocol forced a thirsty rat to consider two potential strategies for discovery, either to heed the light as meaningful or to disregard it–if the latter option were chosen, in the presence of hippocampal damage, the rat reveals an impaired ability to determine what's invariant in space.

If, when we use the word "place," we start thinking about a neural mechanism involved in checking *for what doesn't change* either in time *or* space, then we better understand contemporary hippocampal research, which, ironically, remains interested in engrams of a sort.

* * *

The CA1 neurons that fire when a freely moving rat passes a particular position of space have been termed place cells.

8

Grid and Place

Visiting a foreign school several years ago, I taught neuroanatomy to students, trainees, and faculty–all at the same time (the lectures were in English). A problem in planning was: what level of detail does one deliver in any language to an audience of mixed expertise?

Lecturing on hippocampus and its connections, I thought one could profitably focus on *entorhinal cortex.*

In this monograph, we've described it at various points in chapters four through six. To summarize:

1. Entorhinal cortex is the only unambiguously six-layered structure in the hippocampal formation. It's not archipallium.
2. Entorhinal fibers pass through parasubiculum, presubiculum, subiculum, then across hippocampal fissure/sulcus to dentate gyrus (molecular layer) via the perforant pathway.
3. Entorhinal cortex receives significant input from CA1 and subiculum, but not exclusively from CA1 and subiculum.
4. Entorhinal cortex projects to dentate, CA3, CA1, and subiculum also via perforant pathway.

We're accustomed to thinking about neocortex connecting to other neocortex or about how neocortex projects, say, to spinal cord in a corticospinal tract. But entorhinal cortex linking to hippocampus complex is flat-out peculiar.

Entorhinal cortex is "the primary interface for information flow" between neocortex and the hippocampal complex; neocortical afferents to entorhinal cortex largely arise from cortical (multi-modal) association areas that occupy swaths of surface in primate and human brains (Insausti and Amaral, 2008).

Why does so much cortical information *funnel* to hippocampus? And why does CA1 and subicular output pass back to entorhinal cortex, running opposite to the direction of the funnel's flow?

* * *

Pause for thought.

Last chapter, we mentioned increased firing of certain CA1 neurons when a freely moving rat passed a particular position of space. Thinking for a moment about the receptive field of that place cell: in what possible way does it have any clue about a position in some box, either place or cue? Is a place determined by visual, tactile, olfactory data or by some associative combination of sensations?

History helps us again. Here's a snippet published in 2012: "[T]he source and nature of the inputs to the place cells remained mysterious for several decades. . . . However, a very simple experiment changed the picture. Brun et al. (2002) severed the connections between CA3 and CA1, which left direct input from the entorhinal cortex as the only major cortical input to CA1. . . The strong prediction based on the intrahippocampal models at the time was that spatially modulated firing in CA1 should disappear almost completely. Remarkably, place cells in the lesion group were virtually indistinguishable from place cells in control rats. These results suggested that the spatial signal is computed independently of the intrinsic loop of the hippocampus . . ." (Rowland et al., 2012).

"Computed independently" doesn't mean that dentate and CA3 aren't normally involved in the firing activity of CA1 neurons; but entorhinal cortex and CA1 linked *only* to each other results in place cell firing in CA1 nevertheless. It turns out that place-specific firing has been observed in all subfields of the hippocampus, including dentate gyrus, CA3, and CA1 (Treves et al., 2008).

A reasonable surmise would be that entorhinal cortex conveys information about space. So, people interrogated entorhinal cortex to find that its projection neurons "exhibit sharply turned spatial firing, much like place cells in the hippocampus, except that each cell had multiple firing fields" (Moser et al., 2008).

Confused? You needn't be. A place cell (think CA1, a microelectrode in a CA1 pyramidal neuron) fires in a place in a box:

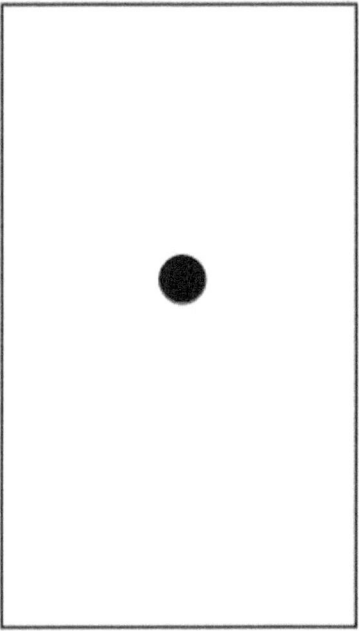

A "grid cell" (think entorhinal cortex, a microelectrode in a projection neuron in a specific layer of entorhinal cortex) fires in many places in a box:

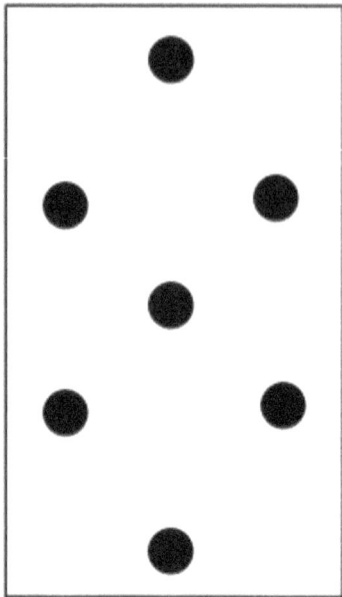

We're talking about just one grid cell in entorhinal cortex. It takes time for an animal to get around in the box. The action potentials of that cell don't fire randomly in the course of travel.

You could change the local environment to discover that grid cells don't "merely mirror sensory stimuli" inside a box (Moser et al., 2008).

I'll rotate the box a few degrees to the right, then 90 degrees to the right.

The grid cell fires in the same positions in space where it fired previously, without reference to the long and short margins of the box:

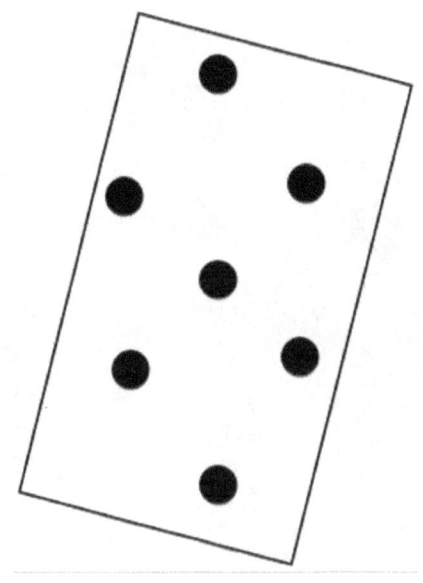

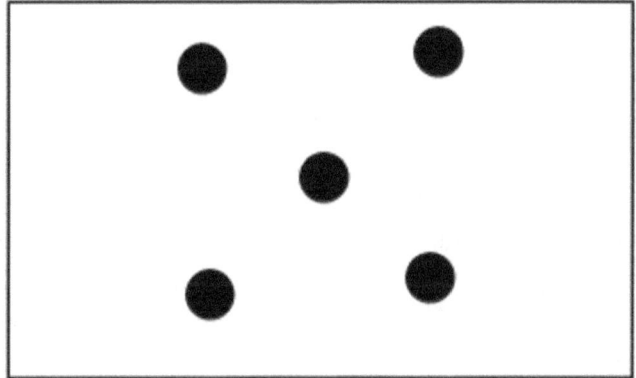

Returning to CA1, even in complete darkness (and independently of the box's orientation, for that matter), a place cell fires in one place:

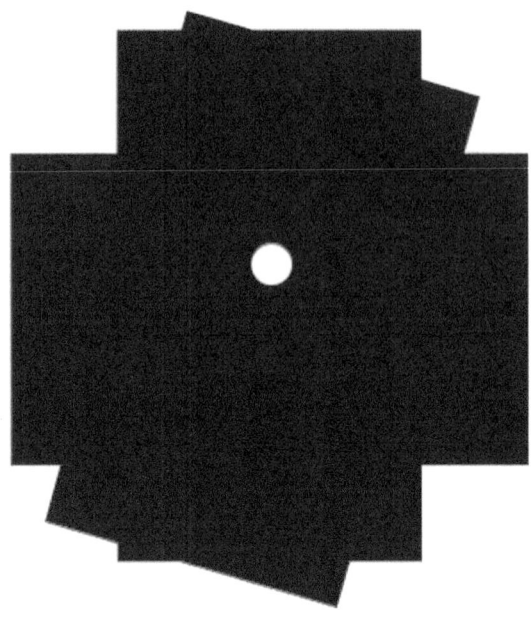

* * *

We should be specific about what it means for a cell "to fire":

> Not only are hippocampal neurons triggered by location cues, but also they respond to salient events in a temporal sequence and nonspatial stimuli such as texture or odors. However, nonspatial variables are not represented by a dedicated subset of neurons or a nonspatial variant of the place cells. . . . [I]n hippocampal cell assemblies, spatial and nonspatial variables (place and color) are represented independently by variation in firing location and firing rate, respectively (Moser et al., 2008).

There are precious times in a career when what one teaches blows one away. A code exists in information processed through connections between entorhinal cortex and hippocampal complex (dentate gyrus and hippocampus proper).

Important in that code are two variables at least: 1. the place/receptive field of the place cell (a WHERE variable, which has to do with location in a grid of the objective environment) and 2. a variable having to do with the rate or perhaps pattern of neural firing (which constitutes an encoded mix of WHERE, WHEN, and WHAT–i.e., WHEN and WHAT carried on the back of a neural representation of an invariant WHERE).

9

Medial Temporal Lobe, A Bit Magnified

Back to anatomy.

But let's not return to human brains immediately.

A first image comes from an astonishing picture book (Retzius, 1906; Taf. LII, figure 5) whose subject is comparative neuroanatomy among species of monkey. The view is of the medial surface of a left chimpanzee hemibrain, with some midline structures dissected away:

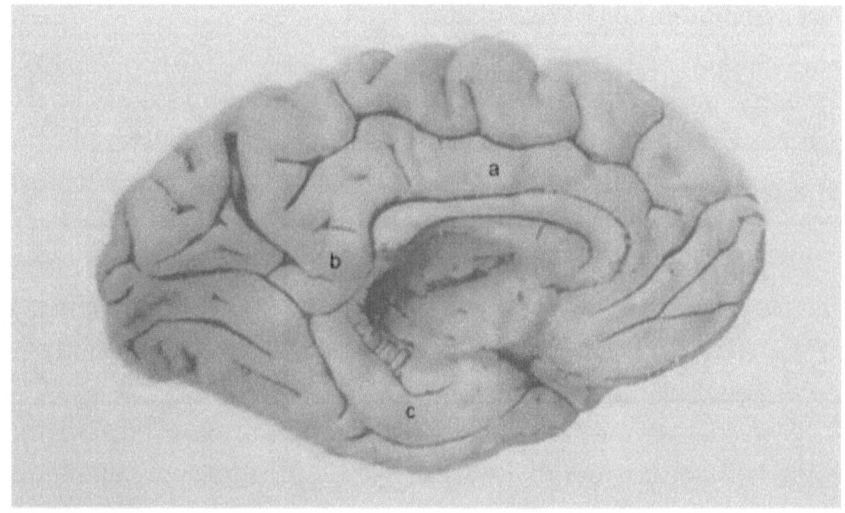

I've labeled three structures, "a," "b," and "c," but my question isn't whether a student can identify them. I'm curious about whether she considers "a, b, and c" to be contiguous. To phrase the question differently, what *is* a gyrus in a brain, such as a putative limbic or paralimbic gyrus?

* * *

The letter labels present difficulties. Am I trying to distinguish anterior (a) and posterior (b) cingulate gyrus–Brodmann areas 24 and 23, respectively–from parahippocampal gyrus (c)? Or does "b" indicate the area of so-called **retrosplenial cortex**–areas 29 and 30? (Some vehemently say that you *never* visualize retrosplenial cortex on any medial surface, because it's buried within the callosal sulcus [Vogt et al., 2000].)

Does cingulate gyrus connect to hippocampus? It's a kind of trick question.

O'Keefe and Nadel (1978a) write that cingulate *just doesn't* project to hippocampus, although to look at a gross specimen, it seems hippocampal complex (dentate gyrus and CA areas) blends eventually into parahippocampal gyrus, and one can follow the latter, in some cases without cortical surface interruption, around the splenium of corpus callosum to the cingulate.

Cingulate gyrus–both anterior and posterior, both with six layers–connects specifically to entorhinal cortex, which also has six layers, not to archipallium directly. It (cingulate) doesn't monosynaptically synapse onto either the dentate gyrus or the proper hippocampus (the CA areas).

Regarding parahippocampal gyrus, which is roughly the area marked both by "c," what part of it do I label? I tried specifically not to encroach upon entorhinal cortex, which is located anteriorly *in* parahippocampal gyrus.

Considering cortical afferents to entorhinal cortex–here's the point–we confuse ourselves when we assume that an anatomic structure, such as parahippocampal gyrus or the vaunted limbic lobe for that matter, is just one entity. It's not.

***

Now consider a human hemibrain's medial surface (right brain, with anterior brain to the left of the image):

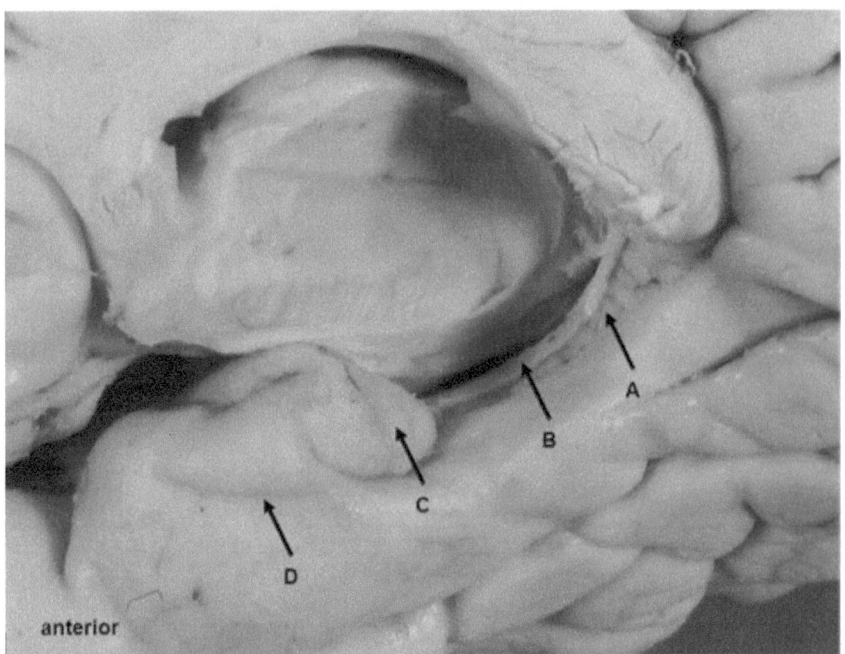

One notices indentations in the area marked by "A," which indicates **dentate gyrus**, whose texture–a **"margo denticulatus"**–lies ventral to **fimbria** (B). The toothy folds mark the course of blood vessels arising either from anterior choroidal artery (a branch of internal carotid) or posterior cerebral artery (specifically, branches of its P2 segment). Both arteries supply much of the hippocampal formation.

A straight, almost vertical bump on the uncus is **the band of Giacomini**, the rostral limit of dentate gyrus; the C arrow points to it.

As we move further anteriorly, we're in an area characterized by significant anatomic variation among individuals, but in most cases (Ovalioglu et al., 2018) we're able to discern a **rhinal sulcus** (arrow D). A view of it becomes clearer if we examine the inferior surface of another brain (we're still looking at right hemibrain; anterior is in the upper part of the picture):

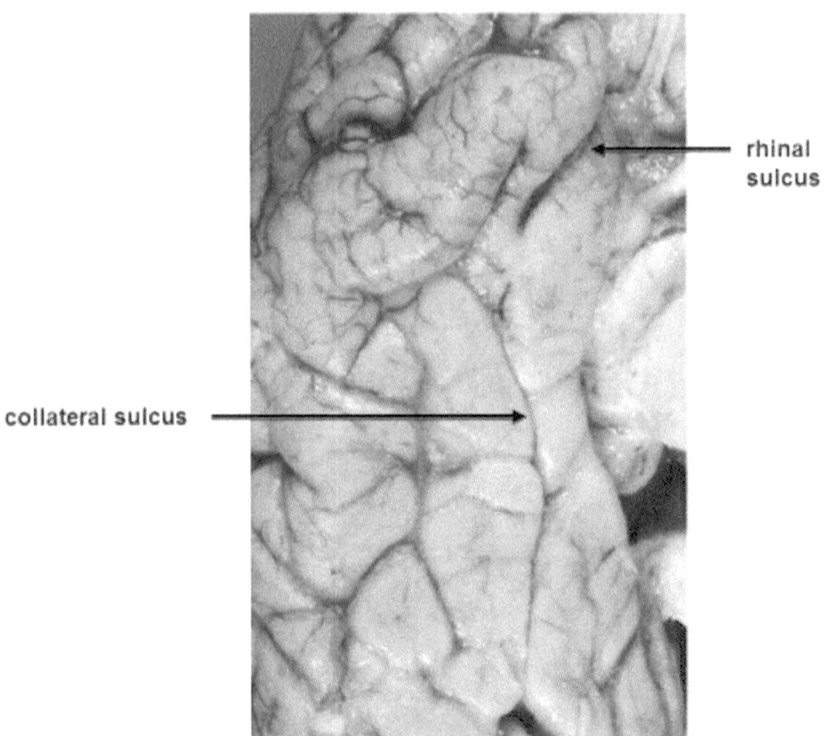

Note that rhinal sulcus is not contiguous with **collateral sulcus**, though it can be as a variant in some brains. Collateral sulcus marks the lateral margin of the parahippocampal gyrus.

Grey matter immediately *lateral* to rhinal sulcus is the territory of Brodmann areas 35 and 36, together known as **perirhinal cortex**. Medial to perirhinal sulcus is domain of **entorhinal cortex** (the best elucidation of both cortical areas in relation to rhinal sulcus is in the macaque monkey [Suzuki and Amaral, 1994]). I won't discuss the several subdivisions of area 36 (which is larger than area

35) or additional parcellations of both parahippocampal gyrus and entorhinal cortex.

* * *

The take home is that parahippocampal gyrus consists, at least, of: 1. perirhinal cortex, 2. entorhinal cortex, and 3. the remainder of a further subdivided parahippocampal gyrus, . . . and there's no direct passage to hippocampus save through those locales. "Previous models of the role of the hippocampus in memory consolidation generally considered the medial temporal lobe as a whole," write Lavenex and Amaral (2000), "and neglected these 'intermediate' cortices (i.e., the entorhinal, perirhinal, and parahippocampal cortices) that were used as mere relays to transfer information from the neocortex to the hippocampus and vice versa." In this chapter, we've mentioned that anterior and posterior cingulate gyrus, Brodmann areas 24 and 23, projects to entorhinal cortex; there are other cortical areas that also do, directly to entorhinal cortex, as we'll summarize in the next chapter), but it's worth noticing that, in essence, we're visualizing a funnel of entry into archipallium. Starting at the top, we have:

Perirhinal Cortex/Parahippocampal Gyrus

Entorhinal Cortex

Hippocampal complex.

Egress out from CA1 in hippocampal complex passes back through the funnel's wide aperture at the top, via subiculum.

10

Negotiating a Triple Entente

In choosing what to read in neuroanatomy, one benefits from two perspectives: the first, a detailed view inside a valley dense with trees and, the second, a vista from some height. Both help us understand the extent of cortical afferents to hippocampus.

Let's look at representative examples of those approaches.

* * *

From Nieuwenhuys et al. (2008, chapter 12):

> The neocortical areas that project directly to the entorhinal cortex include the ventral or agranular insular cortex, the infralimbic cortex (area 25), the caudal orbitofrontal cortex (area 13), the temporopolar cortex (area 38), several fields in the superior temporal gyrus, the prelimbic [frontal, rostral to cingulate gyrus] cortex (area 32), the anterior and posterior cingulate cortex (areas 24 and 23), the dorsolateral prefrontal cortex (areas 9 and 46) and the retrosplenial cortex (areas 29 and 30). . . . [Then, there are specific projections from retrosplenial cortex via parahippocampal gyrus, including, among other areas:] . . . the parietal cortex

(area 7), the occipital cortex (area 19), and the inferior temporal gyrus (area 20).

Unless you have a Brodmann's map in front of you, the above is authoritative but a tad indecipherable.

Note the referenced locales: insula; medial frontal lobe (areas 13, 25, and 32) excluding cingulate gyrus; then cingulate gyrus front, back, as well as retrosplenial cortex; lateral frontal lobe (areas 9 and 46); much of temporal lobe; medial parietal lobe (area 7); and occipital lobe (area 19, a multimodal part of visual cortex).

Much of the multimodal brain, excluding primary sensory or motor cortices, find its way into the area bounded by collateral sulcus.

Nieuwenhuys' valley is replete with detail. It's a thickly settled dale.

Cortical afferents, as diverse as they are, only partially contribute to what Papez called a triple entente or the real-time operational outcome of all inputs–the mediation between an internal milieu, monitored by hypothalamus and brainstem; the external world, information about which derives from primary sensory cortices; and, finally, the world of our schemes and plans. Nieuwenhuys says, "Extrinsic inputs, which are presumed to activate and modulate the intrinsic hippocampal circuitry, arise from . . . (1) various cortical areas [see above], (2) the amygdaloid complex [see our chapters two and six], (3) the medial septal-diagonal band [of Broca] complex [in the basal forebrain, connection to which happens via fornix], (4) the thalamus, (5) the supramamillary region [i.e., hypothalamus and (6) monoaminergic cells masses in the brain stem."

* * *

Here's a second perspective.

In a discussion to which we alluded in chapter six, Nauta and Feirtag (1986) talk about the many projections from frontal association cortex (multimodal neocortex) and inferior temporal association cortex (also multimodal) to both amygdala and hippocampus. "Ordinarily," the authors continue, "one thinks of brain function as working from sensory mechanisms inward–as being directed from sensory receptor organs over a sequence of synaptic way stations to sensory cortex," but afferent sensation to entorhinal cortex differs both qualitatively and in terms of directionality (an inside-out perspective rather than the inverse):

> One might call it a repeatedly preprocessed, multisensory representation of the organism's environment. In this domain nothing is unconditional: the perception of the world is biased by physiological needs. One is reminded of a hungry child's visit to a restaurant. Entering, he sees what people have on their plates. Leaving, he sees that the diners also have faces.

As hippocampologists say (Amaral and Lavenex, 2007), "the general rule is that the entorhinal cortex receives input only from cortical regions with demonstrated polysensory convergence."[13] That's fine, but the hungry child's view of the world is interesting in itself, just as thirst in a water-deprived rat colors and drives the experiments described in chapter seven. The child's entrance into the restaurant is an instance of Papez's triple entente. (Also: one just has to love the part about how faces suddenly appear after dinner.)

A mountain-top view espouses how hippocampal processing has to do convergence (a funnel, if one still needs the metaphor)–and not just in anatomical terms. Information must coalesce, too.

* * *

We've returned to the start of this monograph, to the place where the eye is drawn to a darkest black line and, inside the concavity it creates, to many dots that collect into a neater, tighter band.

---

13 The exception, Amaral and Lavenex note, is olfactory/rhinencephalic input, but "whereas in the rat almost the entire entorhinal cortex receives direct input from the olfactory bulb, in the monkey this is restricted to about 10% of the surface area of the entorhinal cortex."

11

The Minimal Requirement

> A minimal logical requirement for a physical theory of associative memory is that there must be some change in the potential for interaction between input and output elements of a system, resulting from use. (McNaughton et al., 1978)

I like papers (also books and lectures) that specify the very least thing that they are trying to accomplish. Then the minimum requirement for the author is to meet her minimal requirement. If accomplished well, then one can say that the paper, book, or lecture has served its nominal purpose. The above epigraph stipulates a requirement, but the authors aren't exactly talking about their own intentions in what they're about to write. They're saying that *any* theory of associative memory has to account for neural change resulting from use. The specifics you can read for yourself. Change *in potential*, interaction *between* input and output, even the pregnant word "some" are details that matter. As it happens, achieving McNaughton et al.'s minimal logical requirement in the case of hippocampal physiology has proven to be quite a story.

I promised at the start of this monograph that I'd avoid discussing structures of nanometer dimension, and, in truth, Bliss and Lømo (1973) had no concept, either in the late 60's or the early 70's, of any such receptors. For the record, the 1973 paper was based partly on work dating to the late 60's. It's a landmark work, admirably straightforward in its method. All they did was stimulate perforant path in anesthetized rabbits and record from the granule cell layer of dentate gyrus. Their volleys were tetanic. They weren't exactly sure what physiologic stimulation of the perforant path was or what it actually accomplished:

> Our experiments show that there exists at least one group of synapses in the hippocampus whose efficiency is influenced by activity which may have occurred several hours previously–a time scale long enough to be potentially useful for information storage. Whether or not the intact animal makes use in real life of a property which has been revealed by synchronous, repetitive volleys to a population of fibers the normal rate and pattern of activity along which are unknown, is another matter.

There's a nice anatomical nuance in how they stimulated perforant path. The perforant path's fibers are most tightly bundled "as if through a bottleneck" at the so-called **angular bundle**, and that's precisely where Bliss and Lømo delivered volleys.

They weren't interested in fleshing out a physical theory of associative memory. Yet they did produce evidence regarding its minimal logical requirement. There was demonstrable change in the interaction between input and output elements of a system, as a result of use. Just to be clear: we'd expect, at any synapse, that output happens as a result of input; but if "in" over time changes the quality or intensity of "out," then the interaction between in and out must have changed–or, potentially, it's subject to other changes.

That Bliss and Lømo describe what we now accept as long-term potentiation isn't quite the story of this chapter. To me the more interesting aspect, because I like history, is that other groups couldn't replicate the findings and, what's more, neither Bliss nor Lømo, either working alone or together, were able to reproduce their own results after publishing them.[14] In the early 1970's, Lømo abandoned the work for good; Bliss let it go for years.

Lømo has written with refreshing candor about his consternation at the time. You can consult his autobiographical accounts (Lømo, 2016 and 2018), but for our purpose I'd reintroduce Donald Hebb's engram quest, which we introduced in chapter seven. To keep things supremely simple, an engram is just a change in a nervous system as a function of experience. Did Bliss and Lømo in 1973 corroborate Hebb in demonstrating that post-synaptic activity of granule cells in the dentate gyrus changes as a result of particular volleys delivered via the perforant path?

Lømo says that he didn't think at all about Hebb:

> Hebb famously hypothesized that coincident pre- and post-synaptic firing strengthens synapses and many have asked why Tim [Bliss] and I did not refer to this hypothesis. I cannot remember being aware of Hebb at the time of our experiments.
>
> . . . Hebb's ideas about coincident pre- and post-synaptic firing and neuronal assemblies (engrams) were prescient and have stood the test of time well. But did he do much more than formalize ideas current at the time, using diagrams and terms like cells A and B acting together, giving his ideas an appearance of rigour? According to Hebb, Pavlov 'formulated a simple rule for the occurrence of learning. Any stimulus that acts repeatedly at the same time as a response will form a connection between the cortical

---

14 Why the results couldn't be reproduced is a bit beyond the scope of this chapter. Lømo himself speculated (a thought not to be dismissed out of hand) that the animals used in his early work were somehow different–less stressed, perhaps (Lømo, 2018). More importantly, long-term potentiation isn't just one phenomenon, because it happens differently depending on where you study even within the hippocampal formation.

cells involved. Subsequently, the stimulus will be sufficient to arouse the response'. This formulation seems not all that different from Hebb's. But, 50 years later, as discoveries were made that provided a mechanistic explanation for the need for coincident activity, Hebb's formulation was picked up, and the term Hebb synapse spread like a meme or virus that made Hebb, or so it seems, a cult figure.

I am puzzled by the reverence accorded to Hebb (Lømo, 2018).

We shouldn't dismiss Lømo as grumpy; watch YouTube segments of him–he seems humble, affable, even ebullient, despite his age. We might even want to meet the man for a long, candid chat. He's skeptical about what has been called the "rehebbilitation" of memory neuroscience. He reminds us that neither Hebb nor even Pavlov offers data to demonstrate neural or synaptic change having to do with memory. Maybe, as mentioned in chapter four, neurogenesis that happens in dentate gyrus could be physical evidence for a theory of memory in life.

Lømo would say, "maybe not." He could be dead right; at least, he's being scientific.

So, we continue to search *for change in the potential for interaction between input and output elements of a system.*

* * *

Anatomy is all well and good; unavoidably, it's prerequisite in medical and neuroscientific training. But with the minimal logical requirement in mind (for a *physical* theory), how do we visualize how "some" neuronal change transpires in anatomy?

We could just think about volleys into the granule cell layer. I'm about to describe the associative nature of post-synaptic potentiation (McNaughton et al., 1977; McNaughton et al., 1978; Levy and

Steward, 1979; and Nicoll et al., 1988, especially figure 3), but the main concept is input modifying output.

Bliss and Lømo observed that strong input can result in a potentiated output, what's been called a strengthened synapse. In the following discussion, think about only one output neuron.

A single synapse can't be judged to be strong under a microscope, perhaps. But maybe improved synaptic efficiency connotes strength of an association—not just the association of one input to an output.

Let's add another input to the output neuron, but it's a weak one.

Weak input doesn't result in potentiated output from the one neuron.

So what's the value of potentiated output after a strong input?

If weak input happens *at the same time* as strong input, then weak input potentiates output. There's not as much augmentation as with strong input, but a potentiation happens nevertheless.

*	*	*

A student asks—actually, the question has come up many times from more than one student: how do you know that the weak input's effect on output has changed, if you're just measuring output? Answer: you wouldn't necessarily, unless you knew that weak and strong inputs were happening at the same time.

Now comes an even better question (Nicoll et al., 1988): "How does the strong input communicate to the weak input?"

Up until now, we haven't mentioned that inputs could or needed to communicate with each other. But isn't the point of neurons to communicate in the first place? I'll borrow from Nicoll et al. one last time; they're answering their own question about how inputs communicate:

> . . . it is unlikely that some factor can diffuse from the strong synapse to the weak one, either extracellularly or intracellularly. Since the only obvious anatomical structure that bridges the strong

and weak input is the postsynaptic neuron, the site of the association [between strong and weak inputs] is likely the postsynaptic membrane.

To extend my response to the student's question, you wouldn't know about the temporal coincidence of inputs except that potentiation after the weak input persists for a long time–*only* after the coincidence of weak and strong inputs.

In the 1973 paper, the "long time" was the duration of the experiment, about six hours, though persisting effects are now known to last weeks. Lømo adds the nuance that "'postsynaptic firing', as in Hebb's model, isn't necessary for an increase in synaptic efficiency. What is required is coincident pre-synaptic firing and post-synaptic depolarization (Lømo, 2018)." (So, output isn't necessarily an action potential. It could just be an enhanced excitatory post-synaptic potential.)

Given the convergence of cortical inputs described in our chapter ten, does coincidence detection allow for more efficient communication between inputs?

Strength of an association, we said, isn't just the facilitated relationship between one input and one output. A physical change that we might conceptualize, only in the mind's eye (in 2019, as I write–but the future will deliver real-time images, I envision), is a demonstrable increase in associations or connections between inputs.

12

More On Convergence

Fair warning: this chapter is speculative more than anatomic.
It begins with a remembrance.
A late professor of mine, who was iconoclastic and reliably–if not preternaturally–articulate, wrote in 2012:

> Memory, the ability to register, retain, and recall information, is often treated as if it were a tangible entity–a thing capable of being divided into multiple pieces. So we have categories of memory, often composed of pairs of opposites: recent and remote, long term and short term, retrospective and prospective, early and late, explicit and implicit, episodic and semantic, declarative and procedural, recognition and recall, cognitive and perceptual, process and content, working and reference, selectional and instructional, verbal and nonverbal, general and specific, taxon and locale, and still more (Locke, 2012).

You'd have to have known him yourself to glean that, if he were to speak the above paragraph to you in person, he would do so with a streak of humor in riffing all the pairs.

In heaping them one on top of the another, he makes you want to conclude with him that the whole lot is absurd: "With so many binary distinctions, one cannot help but feel there is something wrong, and look around for some other, perhaps more rational approach."

* * *

Whenever he spoke, at a weekly case conference for example, no one ever said a word during or after him. Dead silence was his *doppelgänger*. He'd routinely apologize after extemporaneous speech that could last 20 minutes or more. He spoke in complete paragraphs.

Then an apology took a generic form: "I'm sorry, but why is it that no one says anything?" He wore huge, black-rimmed glasses. His suits (he always wore suits) were a bit tight on him. He clipped his narrow tie to the placket of his shirt with an actual paper clip.

I lost track of him over the years, but an obituary reads as follows (when he left Boston is unclear): "Simeon was born on April 22, 1926 and passed away on Friday, March 11, 2016. Simeon was a resident of Miami Beach, Florida."

* * *

Memory, he said, entails three actions–not three tangibles, since memory itself isn't tangible at all, unlike objects that we touch in space or time.

In remembering, you encode, you store, you retrieve.

Of these constituent processes, arguably all are made possible because of redundant hippocampal circuits in the manner of so-called attractor dynamics. The idea isn't mine; it's been advanced by Moser et al. (2008), but I need help with definitions. For example, what is an "attractor" or, more specifically, an attractor network that's dynamic?

Scholarpedia helps me (http://www.scholarpedia.org/article/Attractor_network): "an attractor network is a network of nodes (i.e., neurons in a biological network), often recurrently connected, whose time dynamics settle to a stable pattern. That pattern may be stationary, time-varying (e.g. cyclic), or even stochastic-looking (e.g., chaotic). The particular pattern a network settles to is called its 'attractor'."

We've laid out an anatomy of recurrent connection in previous chapters, but now comes a *coup de grâce* of insight:

> On the basis of the extensive intrinsic connectivity and modifiability of the CA3 network, theoretical work has indicated attractor dynamics as a potential mechanism for low-interference storage of arbitrary input patterns to the hippocampus. In networks with discrete attractor states (a Hopfield network), associative connections would allow stored memories to be recalled from degraded versions of the original input (pattern completion) without mixing up the memory with other events stored in the network (pattern separation) (Moser et al., 2008).

The passage can be unpacked by focusing on a selected few words in it.

Low-interference storage assumes encoding that, also, isn't compromised by interference or noise. One must first register in order to remember: given errant registry, due to inattention or whatever, then faulty recollection results, by definition.

Degradation, if we're honest about it, is inherent in memory, though we're often predisposed to congratulate ourselves that some memories couldn't possibly degrade over time. Retrieval, in turn, runs the risk of *mix up*. There's entropic uncertainty at play. Contemporary information theory at its most basic demythologizes what information, in the first place, really is: ". . . *information* is sometimes associated with the idea of *knowledge* through its popular use rather than with *uncertainty* and the resolution of uncertainty . . ." (Pierce, 1961, his italics).

A *Hopfield network* (I'll try not to degrade too much of what a Hopfield network really is in the eyes of an expert) resolves a problem of incomplete information by minimizing uncertainty. To do so, in neuronal/cellular terms, means that some invariance in a system—some *stability* (of place, for example)—aides in achieving coherence or correlation between parts or even a large territory of the brain.

Both Hopfield (1982) and his intellectual precursor (Little, 1974) write in mathematical language far beyond my ability to understand either of them fully. Yet, as a neurologist, I have a clinical sense of the problem they and others wrestle (Hebb—whom we mentioned in chapter seven and the previous chapter—among them).

Memory will be lousy if encoding is lousy. Even if encoding is decent, memory can still be lousy, because memories (1.) degrade and (2.) because memories mix, even in normal memory. *Pattern completion* and *pattern separation* are two ways to resolve uncertainty, though the uncertainty never vanishes to zero, even in the absence of disease.

No one really knows today (in 2019) whether encoding, storage, and retrieval are essentially or exclusively hippocampal operations. But hippocampal anatomy, if we review it over and over again, points us to its own recurrent connections at very least. A reason to study hippocampus anatomically is to put actual flesh to the notion of a Hopfield network—or maybe strike "Hopfield" and replace with "redundant-mnemonic."

* * *

A last comment.

In chapter four, I cleared my desk to read Treves et al., 2008. Honest: I did clear my usually too cluttered desk.

If I may opine, *all* the references listed in my bibliography make up a quite decent reading list regarding this monograph's topic, but Treves et al. have us think especially hard about the "darkest black line" that first drew attention in our introductory first chapter.

Especially in their 2008 paper(s) (Moser et al., 2008 is a companion piece, quite beautifully written, and maybe even better than Treves et al., 2008), they're all curious about the fate of what they call "fresh" information and the often irksome, but inevitably encountered interference of prior memory traces:

> . . . conflicting requirements favor separating *anatomically* the afferent inputs operating at storage and at retrieval, to optimize the respective parameters separately. . . . The DG [dentate gyrus] essentially duplicates, with its MF [mossy fiber] projections to CA3, the message that the direct perforant path inputs convey to CA3, about the same patterns of activity in layer II of entorhinal cortex, but it implements the option for anatomical separation. If a new discrete pattern of entorhinal activity has to be stored in CA3, it can first be recoded as a pattern of activity in the DG, and then be transformed by the MF projections into yet another, apparently random, CA3 pattern of activity.

Hippocampal anatomy seems conducive to pattern separation. I think hippocampal anatomy (all that we've discussed thus far, with accompanying pictures and such) could be a collective instrument of pattern completion as well.

If any memory is incomplete, poorly encoded, or eventually degraded, isn't the first task in correcting the problem–the uncertainty in a memory–a matter of repeating the initial data set, if possible?

If a message worthy of remembering doesn't come through on first pass, don't we naturally ask, "um, sorry, could you repeat that?"

How far apart are pattern separation and completion, really?

And, I wonder, can anyone show me a place, anatomically, where redundancy of connections–a checking mechanism, in essence, with stem cells in the vicinity, no less–is as robust?

13

A Parting List

Perhaps uniquely in the history of anatomical terminology, the hippocampus has been associated with a bewildering array of creatures, parts of creatures, or imaginary beasts. A short list would include: a seahorse, a white silk worm, a dolphin, a horse-caterpillar, a sea serpent, a river horse (hippopotamus), ram's horns like those on the head of the Egyptian God Amun (hence "Cornu Ammonis") protecting the Pharaoh Taharqa in the temple of Kawa (the temple once in Sudan), the spur of a rooster's foot, the claw of a raptor, or the "whorled chambered shells of a fossil genus of Cephalopods" (Lewis, 1923 and Pearce, 2001). A ram's horn adorns the cover of this book.

In the preceding twelve chapters, we've mentioned many names associated with the hippocampus in human neuroanatomy. The list isn't too bewildering. As a public service and parting gesture, I reproduce the especially pertinent terms, more or less in the order of their appearance:

hippocampal complex
hippocampus proper
hippocampal formation
allocortex or heterogenetic cortex
archipallium

paleopallium
rhinencephalon
pallium or "a cloak"
corpus callosum
cingulate gyrus
cingulate sulcus
callosal sulcus
hippocampal fissure/sulcus
mammillary body
mammillothalamic tract or the fasciculus of Vicq d'Azyr
anterior nucleus of thalamus
nerves of Lancisi
indusium griseum or the supracallosal hippocampal rudiment
gyrus fasciolaris or fasciola cinerea
taenia tecta
sulcus paraolfactorius posterior
suprapyramidal blade
granule cell layer
molecular layer
hilus
subgranular zone
polymorphic layer, sometimes considered synonymous with "hilus"
mossy-fiber pathway
mossy cells
pyramidal neurons
Cornu Ammonis (CA) or Ammon's horn
"greater limbic system"
regio inferior, a specific part of Cornu Ammonis otherwise known as CA3
regio superior, considered equivalent to CA1
presubiculum
subiculum
parasubiculum
entorhinal cortex
parahippocampal gyrus

entorhinal verrucae
Schaffer collaterals
alveus (belly)
fimbria fornicis (the "fringe" of the fornix)
fornix
fornical or hippocampal commissure.
pre-commissural fornix (anterior to anterior commissure)
post-commissural fornix
nuclei of the septal area
lateral septum
diagonal band of Broca
bed nucleus of the anterior commissure
nucleus accumbens septi
fascicles of Zuckerkandel
medial forebrain bundle
lateral hypothalamus
anteroventral and anteromedial thalamic nuclei (subparts of anterior thalamic nucleus)
mammillo-tegmental tract
postsubiculum (dorsal aspect of presubiculum)
le grand lobe de l'ourlet or the great lobe of the hem
le grand lobe limbique
stria terminalis
amygdalofugal pathway
inferior temporal cortex
place cell
grid cell
anterior and posterior cingulate gyrus (Brodmann areas 24 and 23, respectively)
retrosplenial cortex (Brodmann areas 29 and 30)
margo denticulatus
anterior choroidal artery (a branch of internal carotid)
posterior cerebral artery (specifically, branches of its P2 segment)
the band of Giacomini (an almost vertical bump on the uncus)
rhinal sulcus

collateral sulcus
perirhinal cortex (Brodmann areas 35 and 36)
insula
medial frontal lobe (Brodmann areas 13, 25, and 32)
lateral frontal lobe (Brodmann areas 9 and 46)
medial parietal lobe (Brodmann area 7)
occipital lobe (Brodmann area 19, a multimodal part of visual cortex)
angular bundle

The observant student will note that I left **dentate gyrus** off the list, even though it was among the first structures we described. The reason is personal. After all these years, it still strikes me as more wondrous than its name.

REFERENCES

Permission to reproduce anatomical images is gratefully acknowledged from two sources. Images on pages 2, 24, 25, 61, and 62 are reproduced from Joseph and Cardozo, 2004, with permission from John Wiley and Sons, Inc. Images on pages 19 and 31 are reproduced with permission from the Michigan State University Brain Biodiversity Bank, supported by the National Science Foundation.

On page 41, permission to modify and reproduce a diagram from Edlow et al., 2016 has been granted by Mary Ann Liebert, Inc.

Books and Monographs
Anderson, Per, Morris, Richard, Amaral, David, Bliss, Tim, and O'Keefe, John, eds. *The Hippocampus Book*. New York and Oxford: Oxford University Press, 2007.

Beach, Frank A., Hebb, Donald O., Morgan, Clifford T., Nissen, Henry W., eds. *The Neuropsychology of Lashley. Selected Papers of K.S. Lashley*. New York, Toronto, London: McGraw-Hill, 1960.

Brodal, Alf. *Neurological Anatomy In Relation to Clinical Medicine* [3rd ed.]. New York and Oxford: Oxford University Press, 1981.

Carpenter, Malcolm B. and Sutin, Jerome. *Human Neuroanatomy* [8th ed.]. Baltimore and London: Williams and Wilkins, 1983.

Crosby, Elizabeth C and Schnitzlein, H. N., eds. *Comparative Correlative Neuroanatomy of the Vertebrate Telencephalon*. New York: MacMillan, 1982.

Duvernoy, Henri M. *The Human Hippocampus. Functional Anatomy, Vascularization and Serial Sections with MRI* [3rd ed.]. Berlin, Heidelberg, New York: Springer-Verlag, 2005.

Farah, Martha J. *Visual Agnosia. Disorders of Object Recognition and What They Tell Us about Normal Vision.* Cambridge and London: MIT Press, 1990.

Good, Byron J. *Medicine, Rationality, and Experience: An Anthropological Perspective.* Cambridge and New York: Cambridge University Press, 1993.

Hebb, D.O. *The Organization of Behavior. A Neuropsychological Theory* [Reprint]. Mahwah, New Jersey and London: Lawrence Erlbaum, 2002, original publication in 1949.

Johnston, J.B. *The Nervous System of Vertebrates.* London: John Murray, 1907.

Joseph, Jeffrey T. and Cardozo, David L. *Functional Neuroanatomy. An Interactive Text and Manual.* Hoboken: John Wiley and Sons, 2004.

Llinás, Rodolfo R. *I of the Vortex. From Neurons to Self.* Cambridge and London: MIT Press, 2001.

Locke, Simeon. *Seven Kine, Fatfleshed. A Theory of Sleep and Dreams.* No publication city: Xlibris, 2012.

Luria, A.R. *The Working Brain. An Introduction to Neuropsychology.* Trans. Basil Haigh. New York: Basic Books, 1973.

Luria, Aleksandr Romanovich. *Higher Cortical Functions in Man.* [2nd ed.]. Trans. Basil Haigh. New York: Basic Books, 1980.

Nauta, Walle J.H. and Feirtag, Michael. *Fundamental Neuroanatomy.* New York: W.H. Freeman, 1986.

Nieuwenhuys, Rudolf, Voogd, Jan, van Huijzen Chrisitaan. *The Human Central Nervous System* [4th ed.]. Berlin, Heidelberg, New York: Springer-Verlag, 2008.

Nolte, John. *The Human Brain. An Introduction to Its Functional Anatomy* [4th ed]. St. Louis: Mosby, 1999

O'Keefe, John and Nadel, Lynn. *The Hippocampus as a Cognitive Map.* Oxford: Clarendon Press, 1978.

Pierce, J.R. *Symbols, Signals and Noise. The Nature and Process of Communication.* New York: Harper and Row, 1961.

Retzius, Gustaf. *Das Affenhirn in Bildicher Darstellung.* Jena: Gustav Fisher, 1906.

Shepherd, Gordon M., ed. *The Synaptic Organization of the Brain* [4th ed]. New York and Oxford: Oxford University Press, 1998.

Szabo K. and Hennerici M.G., eds. *The Hippocampus in Clinical Neuroscience. Frontiers of Neurology and Neuroscience,* vol. 34. Basel: Karger, 2014.

Tarin, Pierre. *Adversia anatomica, de omnibus corporis humani partium, tum descriptionibus, cum picturis. Adversaria anatomica prima, de omnibus cerebri, nervorum & organorum functionibus animalibus inservientium, descriptionibus & iconismis.* Paris: Moreau, 1750 (persistent URL: https://wellcomelibrary.org/item/b30408234).

Winter, Alison. *Memory. Fragments of a Modern History.* Chicago and London: University of Chicago Press, 2012.

Articles and Specific Chapters in Books

Aimone JB, Deng W, Gage FH. Resolving new memories: a critical look at the dentate gyrus, adult neurogenesis, and pattern separation. *Neuron* 2011;70:589-596.

Amaral D and Lavenex P. Hippocampal neuroanatomy. In: *The Hippocampus Book.* New York and Oxford: Oxford University Press, 2007, pp. 37-114.

Andersen P, Morris R, Amaral D, Bliss T, O'Keefe J. Historical perspective: proposed functions, biological characteristics, and neurobiological models of the hippocampus. In: *The Hippocampus Book.* New York and Oxford: Oxford University Press, 2007, pp. 9-36.

Augustinack JC, Helmer K, Huber KE, Kakunoori S, Zöllei L, Fischl B. Direct visualization of the perforant pathway in the human brain with *ex vivo* diffusion tensor imaging. *Frontiers in Human Neuroscience* 2010, doi: 10.3389/fnhum.2010.00042.

Augustinack JC, Huber KE, Postelnicu GM, Frosch MP, Pienaar R, Fischl B. Entorhinal verrucae correlate with surface geometry. *Translational Neuroscience* 2012;3:123-131.

Bir SC, Ambekar S, Kukreja S, Nanda A. Julius Caesar Arantius (Guilio Cesare Aranzi, 1530-1589) and the hippocampus of the human brain: history behind the discovery. *Journal of Neurosurgery* 2015;122:971-975.

Bliss TVP and Lømo T. Long-lasting potentiation of synaptic transmission in the dentate area of the anesthetized rabbit following stimulation of the perforant path. *Journal of Physiology* 1973;232:331-356.

Boring EG. Introduction. Lashley and cortical integration. In: *The Neuropsychology of Lashley. Selected Papers of K.S. Lashley.* New York, Toronto, London: McGraw-Hill, 1960, pp. xi-xvi.

Braford MR. Comparative aspects of forebrain organization in the ray-finned fishes: touchstones or not? *Brain, Behavior and Evolution* 1995;46:259-274.

Brodal A. The olfactory pathways. The amygdala. The hippocampus. The limbic system. In: *Neurological Anatomy In Relation to Clinical Medicine* [3rd ed.]. New York and Oxford: Oxford University Press, 1981, especially pp. 673-697.

Brun VH, Otnæss MK, Molden S, Steffenach H-A, Witter MP, Moser M-B, Moser EI. Place cells and place recognition by direct entorhinal-hippocampal circuitry. *Science* 2002;296:2243-2246.

Butler AB. Of horse-caterpillars and homologies: evolution of the hippocampus and its name. *Brain, Behavior and Evolution* 2017;90:7-14.

Catani M, Dell'Acqua F, Thiebaut de Schotten M. A revised limbic system model for memory, emotion and behaviour. *Neuroscience and Biobehavioral Reviews* 2013;37:1724-1737.

Di Ieva A, Fathalla H, Cusimano MD, Tschabitscher M. The indusium griseum and the longitudinal striae of the corpus callosum. *Cortex* 2015;62:34-40.

Di Ieva A, Tschabitscher M, Rodriguez y Baena R. Lancisi's nerves and the seat of the soul. *Neurosurgery* 2007;60:563-568.

Edlow BL, McNab JA, Witzel T, Kinney HC. The structural connectome of the human central homeostatic network. *Brain Connectivity* 2016;6:187-200.

Farah MJ. Interpreting the associative agnosias in terms of theories of normal object recognition. In: *Visual Agnosia. Disorders of Object Recognition and What They Tell Us about Normal Vision.* Cambridge and London: MIT Press, 1990, pp. 93-143.

Gage FH. Mammalian neural stem cells. *Science* 2000;287:1433-1438.

Golgi C. History of Neuroscience. On the fine structure of the pes Hippocampi major (with plates XIII-XXIII) [Trans. Bentivoglio M and Swanson LW]. *Brain Research Bulletin* 2001;54:461-483.

Good BJ. How medicine constructs its object. In: *Medicine, Rationality, and Experience: An Anthropological Perspective.* Cambridge and New York: Cambridge University Press, 1993, pp. 65-87.

Haberly LB. Olfactory Cortex. In: *The Synaptic Organization of the Brain.* Ed. Shepherd GM. New York: Oxford, 1998, pp. 377-416.

Hebb DO. Studies in the organization of behavior. I. Behavior of the rat in a field orientation. *Journal of Comparative Psychology* 1938a;25:333-352.

Hebb DO. Studies in the organization of behavior. II. Changes in the field orientation of the rat after cortical destruction. *Journal of Comparative Psychology* 1938b;26:427-444.

Hebb DO. Perception of a complex: the phase sequence. In: *The Organization of Behavior. A Neuropsychological Theory* [Reprint]. Mahwah, New Jersey and London: Lawrence Erlbaum, 2002, original publication in 1949, pp. 79-106.

Hopfield JJ. Neural networks and physical systems with emergent collective computational abilities. *Proceedings of the National Academy of Sciences* 1982;79:2554-2558.

Humphrey T. The development of the human hippocampal fissure. *Journal of Anatomy* 1967;101:655-676.

Insausti R and Amaral DG. The entorhinal cortex of the monkey: IV. Topographical and laminar organization of cortical afferents. *Journal of Comparative Neurology* 2008;509:608-641.

Johnston D and Amaral DG. Hippocampus. In: *The Synaptic Organization of the Brain*. Ed. Shepherd GM. New York: Oxford, 1998, pp. 417-458.

Kier EL, Fulbright RK, Bronen RA. Limbic lobe embryology and anatomy: dissection and MR of the medial surface of the fetal cerebral hemisphere. *American Journal of Neuroradiology* 1995;16:1847-1853.

Lavenex P and Amaral DG. Hippocampal-neocortical interaction: a hierarchy of associativity. *Hippocampus* 2000;10:420-430.

Levy WB and Steward O. Synapses as associative memory elements in the hippocampal formation. *Brain Research* 1979;175:233-245.

Lewis FT. The significance of the term *Hippocampus*. *Journal of Comparative Neurology* 1923;35:213-230.

Li G and Pleasure SJ. The development of hippocampal cellular assemblies. *WIREs Developmental Biology* 2014;3:165-177. doi: 10.1002/wdev.127.

Lim C and Alexander MP. Stroke and episodic memory disorders. *Neuropsychologia* 2009;47:3045-3058.

Little WA. The existence of persistent states in the brain. *Mathematical Biosciences* 1974;19:101-120.

Lømo T. Scientific discoveries: what is required for lasting impact. *Annual Review of Physiology* 2016;78:1-21.

Lømo T. Review. Discovering long-term potentiation (LTP)– recollections and reflections on what came after. *Acta Physiologica* 2018;222,doi: 10.1111/apha.12921.

Luria AR. Investigation of mnestic processes. In: *Higher Cortical Functions in Man*. [2nd ed.] Trans. Basil Haigh. New York: Basic Books, 1980, pp. 469-485.

Luria AR. Memory. In: *The Working Brain. An Introduction to Neuropsychology*. Trans. Basil Haigh. New York: Basic Books, 1973, pp. 280-302.

Maguire EA, Burgess N, Donnett JG, Frackowiak RSJ, Frith CD, O'Keefe J. Knowing where and getting there: a human navigation network. *Science* 1998;280:921-924.

McAvoy KM, Scobie KN, Berger S, Russo C, Guo N, Decharatanachart P, Vega-Ramirez H, Miake-Lye S, Whalen M,

Nelson M, Bergami M, Bartsch D, Hen R, Berninger B, Sahay A. Modulating neuronal competition dynamics in the dentate gyrus to rejuvenate aging memory circuits. *Neuron* 2016;91:1356-1373.

McNaughton BL and Barnes CA. Physiological identification and analysis of dentate granule cell responses to stimulation of the medial and lateral perforant pathways in the rat. *Journal of Comparative Neurology* 1977;175:439-454.

McNaughton BL, Douglas RM, Goddard GV. Synaptic enhancement in fascia dentata: cooperativity among coactive afferents. *Brain Research* 1978;157:277-293.

Moser EI. Grid cells and the entorhinal map of space. Nobel Lecture, 7 December 2014, available at www.nobelprize.org.

Moser EI, Kropff E, Moser —B. Place cells, grid cells, and the brain's spatial representation system. *Annual Review of Neuroscience* 2008;31:69-89.

Nicoll RA, Kauer JA, Malenka RC. The current excitement in long-term potentiation. *Neuron* 1988;1:97-103.

Nieuwenhuys R. The development and general morphology of the telencephalon of actinopterygian fishes: synopsis, documentation and commentary. *Brain Structure and Function* 2011;215:141-157.

Northcutt RG. Evolution of the telencephalon in nonmammals. *Annual Review of Neuroscience* 1981;4:301-350.

O'Keefe J. Hippocampal neurophysiology in the behaving animal. In: *The Hippocampus Book*. New York and Oxford: Oxford University Press, 2007, pp. 475-548.

O'Keefe J. Spatial cells in the hippocampal formation. Nobel lecture, 7 December 2014, available at www.nobelprize.org.

O'Keefe J and Dostrovsky J. The hippocampus as a spatial map. Preliminary evidence from unit activity in the freely moving rat. *Brain Research* 1971;34:171-175.

O'Keefe J and Nadel L. Anatomy. In: *The Hippocampus as a Cognitive Map*. Oxford: Clarendon Press, 1978a, pp. 102-140.

O'Keefe J and Nadel L. Introduction to the lesion review. In: *The Hippocampus as a Cognitive Map*. Oxford: Clarendon Press, 1978b, pp. 231-239.

O'Keefe J, Nadel L, Keightley S, Kill D. Fornix lesions selectively abolish place learning in the rat. *Experimental Neurology* 1975;48:152-166.

Ovalioglu AO, Ovalioglu TC, Canaz G, Emel E. Morphologic variations of the collateral sulcus on the mediobasal region of the temporal lobe: an anatomical study. *World Neurosurgery* 2018;118:e212-e216. doi: 10.1016/j.wneu.2018.06.156.

Papez, JW. A proposed mechanism of emotion. *Archives of Neurology and Psychiatry* 1937a;38:725-743, reprinted in Neylan TC [section ed.]. Neuropsychiatry classics. A proposed mechanism of emotion. *Journal of Neuropsychiatry and Clinical Neurosciences* 1995;7:103-112.

Papez JW. The brain considered as an organ: neural systems and central levels of organization. *American Journal of Psychology* 1937b;49:217-232.

Pearce JMS. Ammon's horn and the hippocampus. *Journal of Neurology, Neurosurgery and Psychiatry* 2001;71:351.

Rasonja MB, Orešković D, Knezović V, Pogledić I, Pupačić D, Vukšić M, Brugger PC, Prayer D, Petanjek Z, Milošević NJ. Histological and MRI study of the development of the human indusium griseum. *Cerebral Cortex* 2019;doi: 10.1093/cercort/bhz004bhz004.

Rodríguez F, López JC, Vargas JP, Broglio C, Gómez Y, Salas C. Spatial memory and hippocampal pallium through vertebrate evolution: insights from reptiles and teleost fish. *Brain Research Bulletin* 2002;57:499-503.

Rowland DC, Roudi Y, Moser M-B, Moser EI. Ten years of grid cells. *Annual Review of Neuroscience* 2016;39:19-40.

Salas C, Broglio C, Rodriguez F. Evolution of forebrain and spatial cognition in vertebrates: conservation across diversity. *Brain, Behavior and Evolution* 2003;62:72-82.

Scoville WB and Milner B. Loss of recent memory after bilateral hippocampal lesions. *Journal of Neurology, Neurosurgery, and Psychiatry* 1957;20:11-21.

Showers MJC. Telencephalon of birds. In: *Comparative Correlative Neuroanatomy of the Vertebrate Telencephalon*. Eds. Crosby EC and Schnitzlein HN. New York: MacMillan, 1982, pp. 218-246.

Suzuki WA and Amaral DG. Perirhinal and parahippocampal cortices of the macaque monkey: cortical afferents. *Journal of Comparative Neurology* 1994;350:497-533.

Tatu L and Vuillier F. Structure and vascularization of the hippocampus. In: *The Hippocampus in Clinical Neuroscience. Frontiers of Neurology and Neuroscience*, vol. 34. Eds. Szabo K. and Hennerici M.G. Basel: Karger, 2014, pp. 18-25.

Toni N and Schindler AF. Maturation and functional integration of new granule cells into the adult hippocampus. *Cold Spring Harbor Perspectives in Biology* 2016;8:a018903.

Treves A, Tashiro A, Witter MP, Moser EI. Forefront review. What is the mammalian dentate gyrus good for? *Neuroscience* 2008;154:1155-1172.

Vargas JP, Bingman VP, Portavella M, López JC. Telencephalon and geometric space in goldfish. *European Journal of Neuroscience* 2006;24:2870-2878.

Vogt BA, Absher JR, Bush G. Human retrosplenial cortex: where is it and is it involved in emotion [letter]. *Trends in Neurosciences* 2000;23:195-196.

Winter A. Wilder Penfield and the recording of personal experience. In: *Memory. Fragments of a Modern History*. Chicago and London: University of Chicago Press, 2012, pp.75-102.

Wyss JM and Sripanidkulchai K. The indusium griseum and anterior hippocampal continuation in the rat. *Journal of Comparative Neurology* 1983;219:251-272.

Zeidman P and Maguire EA. Anterior hippocampus: the anatomy of perception, imagination, and episodic memory. *Nature Reviews Neuroscience* 2016;17:173-182.

www.ingramcontent.com/pod-product-compliance
Lightning Source LLC
Chambersburg PA
CBHW021452210526
45463CB00002B/746